Coping with Color-Blindness

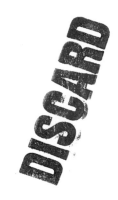

Coping
with Color-Blindness

Odeda Rosenthal
Robert H. Phillips, PhD

Avery Publishing Group

Garden City Park, New York

The medical and psychological information and suggestions presented in this book are not intended as a substitute for consulting your physician or mental-health professional. All matters concerning your physical health should be supervised by a medical professional.

Cover design: William Gonzalez and Rudy Shur
In-house editor: Karen Hay
Typesetter: Elaine V. McCaw
Printer: Paragon Press, Honesdale, PA

Avery Publishing Group
120 Old Broadway
Garden City Park, Ny 11040
1-800-548-5757

Cataloging-in-Publication Data

Rosenthal, Odeda
  Coping with colorblindness : sound helpful strategies & advice
for those who must deal with inherited or acquired color vision
confusion / Odeda Rosenthal.
  p. cm.
  Includes bibliographical references and index.
  ISBN 0-89529-733-7

  1. Color blindness. I. Title.

RE921.R68 1997   617.7'59
                      QB197-40335

10 9 8 7 6 5 4 3 2 1

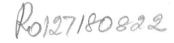

Table of Contents

Acknowledgements

Thanks are due the many men and women of all ages and backgrounds who have colorblindness, whether inherited or acquired, who have helped to explain the problem. Their encouraging words and their willingness to have their cases published are most appreciated.

Thanks also go to Judith E. Gurland, M.D., assistant director of ophthalmology at Bronx-Lebanon Hospital Center and senior pediatric ophthalmologist at Montefiore Hospital, Bronx, New York, who encouraged the writing of this book; to Diane Simpson Milenic of the National Institutes of Health, who scouted to bring to light the most current publications on the subject; to Elizabeth Tunis, the librarian at the National Library of Medicine who pointed out historical material; to the many librarians of medical schools, university libraries, especially the libraries of East Carolina University and its School of Medicine, the Library of Congress, the New York School of Optometry, and others who helped with the research.

Some of the material was first published in *Computer Graphics Magazine*, *More Magazine* (New Zealand), *Christchurch Press* (New Zealand), *Globe and Mail* (Canada), *Adult And Continuing Education Today*, *East Hampton Star*, *Optics and Photonics News*, and in the proceedings of the International Computer Color Graphics Conference (Tallahassee, Florida, 1983), Compint, the International Computer Technologies Conference (Montreal, Canada, 1985), the National Computer Graphics Association Conference (Anaheim, California, 1988) and the OPTCON conference of the Optical Society of America (San Jose, California, 1991).

And thanks to the author-neurologist Dr. Oliver Sacks, to the pioneer vision scientist Dr. Jay Neitz, and to the cognitive psychologist who specializes in the psychophysics of vision, Dr. Leo Hurvich, for each of their personal insights and interest in my effort to explain this complex topic to the general public as I focus on the human factor—real cases.

Thanks to Harlan A. Rosenthal, a computer systems engineer, who happens to be my son. From the early days of the computer graphics industry in the 1970s, he urged that I speak up, especially since he noted that much of the early work was done by physicists, mathematicians, and others who were not well-versed in cognitive studies, and as he also noted, were often colorblind. His professional and personal critical analysis of my work and warm support through the years is most appreciated.

Karen Hay, senior editor of this volume, was instrumental in whipping it into shape, and making it a reality at long last. Heartfelt thanks are due to her.

Last but not least, thanks to Alexander M. Milenic and Lorelle Fallon (whose son is colorblind), and to my daughter Heidi Rosenthal Vincent and Bette Roy (whose husband is colorblind) for reading portions of the manuscript to assure that the general reader would find it clear and useful.

Preface

Two hundred years ago, the distinguished British scientist John Dalton published the first significant explanation of color vision confusion. In fact, he was describing his own condition and that of his brother. One would think that much research and writing on this topic would have been done since that time, but this is not the case. Through the years, I have become increasingly aware of the public's lack of knowledge about colorblindness.

I first became interested in the subject in the 1960s when I taught commercial graphics at DeWitt Clinton High School in the Bronx, which was then a rough, all-boys' school. Although I was preparing students for potential jobs in the real world, to the school counselors, art courses were a way of dealing with trouble makers, a kind of therapy to soothe savage beasts who would not sit still for academic work.

At one point, four boys who were thrown out of shop class landed in my room. What was their crime? It was said that they had been clowning around and causing a dangerous situation.

What had they done? They had caused chaos, I was told, and that had led to fights and fires. They had mixed up electrical wires, causing sparks and blown fuses. Besides causing others to lose electricity, the "clowns" often replaced tools improperly. The tools were supposed to be hung on a board that was painted black and had red numbers corresponding to numbers on the tools. All of this was seen as willful misbehavior on the part of the four boys.

It turned out, however, that the four had not known each other before meeting in shop class. They had not ganged-up to do harm, nor did they discuss among themselves the incidents that occurred. In my art class, the four disruptive students were fine. For the most part, they showed genuine creativity and willingness to follow instructions, to learn, and to complete tasks. Not one ever rebelled even though I was often considered a strict and demanding teacher.

What was the reason for this change of behavior? All four boys were colorblind, which is what I had suspected. Not one had been tested for color vision, and none could accept the idea of being "handicapped" or "blind." But you could see the relief when I explained to each the possible reason for his problems.

I tried to tell career counselors that it was a mistake to assign students to tasks they could not complete because of confused color vision. The counselors assumed I was being soft on the "punks." They saw no reason to test students for color vision. Eventually, I learned to keep my opinions to myself.

But these problems don't go away, nor are they confined to schoolrooms. Time and again, I hear of difficulties among my married friends. Couples argue about decorating new homes and making clothing choices. They often bicker about whether a curtain or a sofa or a dress is one color or another. A wife might ask her husband's advice and he might offer what he considers a grand combination of colors only to be told it is awful. Or she might bow to his opinion and then simply hate being in the house. He might give up and tell his wife she can decorate as she pleases. But she wishes to please him, too. He might suggest she wear something in a color she abhors, or he seems careless in his selection of clothes.

And there are other complaints. Why wasn't he excited about a sunset in a romantic setting? Why couldn't he read a map? The list goes on.

Clearly, colorblindness plays a role in these family feuds, but few consider the possibility that the cause of these color-related arguments could be a genuine physical disorder. Generally, the differing opinions would be seen as a matter of stubbornness or a question of who would get the upper hand. Is the problem worth anger and bitterness?

The problem gets even deeper than marital bickering, sometimes there are legal battles caused by color vision confusion. One day, I was called by an insurance company lawyer who knows that I have a unique perspective on how people perceive things. He needed me to solve a puzzle: Why were there suddenly an overwhelming number of lawsuits against dentists? The health of the insurance company was at stake!

I immediately thought of the new plastic that had been developed to permit capping of teeth at a reasonable price. No longer were beautiful teeth for movie stars only; anyone could now afford to have his or her teeth capped. Those who went to a dentist in quest of the beauty provided by caps first had to have their teeth ground. They had to endure pain and they had to pay for the whole process in order to get compliments. But many did not get compliments. Instead, they were being asked why their teeth had odd colors that didn't match. This made them so furious at the dentists that they sued.

I suggested to the baffled lawyer that the color of the caps might be the problem. Typically, people do not have white teeth. To match the teeth, dentists must select slightly yellow or brownish tones for the caps. These tones are closer to the natural tooth color of most people, which is affected by the foods they eat, the beverages they drink, or the pipes and cigarettes they smoke. Perhaps the dentists being sued were colorblind.

My suggestion was based on a hunch, on observation, and on conversations with some denture specialists who had long been plagued by the problem of matching colors even though their craftsmanship was flawless. Little did I know then, that as early as 1931, the American Dental Association (ADA) had been alerted to the problem of colorblind dentists. At that time, few people were using the services of dentists, so it seemed an insignificant problem.

I made several suggestions to the lawyer about how to deal with the situation. I suggested that patients who sued might be willing to settle for an offer of recapping at no cost, and an assurance that this time, the caps would be selected from a chart by a female dental assistant and a computer color analysis. I was well aware that some females may be colorblind, and that computers are not foolproof. But I also knew at the time, in the early 1970s, that people did not generally know these facts. Their willingness to accept the offer would prove that the dentist was not incompetent, but a poor judge of cap colors. My suggestions worked. They worked so well that New York University's Dental School introduced a required seminar on color vision and its effects on the dental profession, and computerized color-matching is now standard.

My experience with colorblindness hit much closer to home when my husband began to lose color vision as a result of a hypertension medication he was taking in the early 1970s. His loss of color vision was gradual. My husband hesitated to say anything because he was afraid he was going crazy, and he also feared my reaction.

I saw the change for myself. I was well aware of his previous ability to distinguish colors versus his current groping to match suit and tie.

When I asked my husband's doctor if the medicine could cause color vision confusion, he said I should stop being an "overprotective" wife. That's when my research began in earnest.

As a result of that research, which has been going on for more than twenty years, I have spoken at major conferences in the United States and overseas, and published extensively on the subject of colorblindness, or color vision confusion (CVC), as I prefer to call it. In 1985, I was invited to a conference in Canada dealing with computer graphics. At that conference, I said that colorblindness is more hushed up today than homosexuality ever was. I said it was time for the world of technology to consider the problems involved in this form of visual miscommunication.

Why colorblindness has not been dealt with openly is a good question. People in the arts have told me it is a matter for the medical community, and people in medicine think it is of significance only to people in the arts.

One fiber optics expert told me, on the sly, that he deals with audio transmission rather than visual transmission via fiber optics because he cannot see colors properly. His son sees the full range of colors and can hardly believe that his father—a professor with keen eye sight—cannot distinguish one traffic light from another. Pained that even his son does not understand him, the man asked me to explain his problem to the boy. He could not find any information about the subject or the plight of those who deal with it.

Like many others, the professor begged me to write a book that would serve as a general source of information, and to do so using nontechnical language. And so *Coping With Colorblindness* was born.

Coping With Colorblindness attempts to raise consciousness about the significance of color vision confusion by providing information for both the general reader and the specialist. It touches on the various types of colorblindness, the history of color vision research, the causes of colorblindness, colorblindness in women, and the pros and cons of available tests that detect colorblindness. In addition, Dr. Robert Phillips discusses ways of coping with this generally uncorrectable disorder through clearer understanding, humor, positive thinking, relaxation techniques, support groups, and professional assistance.

This book is meant to fill a void, to be a reference for the general reader as well as the specialists. The volume is presented in the hopes that it will offer information, a chuckle, and comfort to all.

Introduction

"God made many beautiful colors. The problem for me is to know what they are and where they are, and how to put them in the right place." These are the words of a man who has inherited colorblindness.

Have you ever considered what life would be like without color? Probably not. But think about it, colors speak to us. They are an important part of our vocabulary of vision. Colors tell us when to stop or go in traffic. They coax us to spend money on clothes. They entice us to eat foods, and cause us to not eat foods. Colors inform us of weather and temperature. A flushed face or sunburned skin can inform us of fever or over-exposure. A grey sky warns us that a storm is coming. Colors help us differentiate between similar looking pills and even our bills. They warn us of danger, and delight our spirits.

Have you ever heard someone say that colors do not matter? That is not true! It would be like saying that rhythm is not important to hearing voices or music. Or that you can assign any rhythm to a line of poetry simply to suit yourself without regard for the poet's intent.

Yes, we do tend to take colors for granted. We tend to minimize their value as a source of information and think of them only in terms of decoration, movie sets, makeup, and moods. There are even people who think that everyone sees colors differently. But then the various colors could not have names assigned to them. And colors are so important in our lives that they have names in all languages. Since biblical days, colors seem to have been a very important part of the lives of people around the world. Remember Joseph and his many-colored dream coat? Various cultures have given colors special significance, even assuming that colors have certain powers and going so far as to forbid some as evil.

In any culture, specific names for colors elicit the same kinds of responses as do other naming words. Consider, for instance, the word "cat." When you hear it, you may not know that it is spelled C-A-T, but you will have the image of a cat in your mind. You may not like cats, or you may love them. You might imagine a cat of one size or another, of one breed or another, of one color or another, but it will definitely be a cat. In no way will you mistake it in your mind for a dog.

This is true of color words as well. Colors trigger certain associations in people's minds. The word green will trigger a particular reaction or association in any person's mind. A green apple will look green to everybody—to everybody, that is, who can see green; there are people who are green colorblind. You may not like the color green, or you may not like to bite into an apple that is green because you assume that it will be sour. Other people may like the color; they may like the taste of tart apples. What the person with green color vision confusion sees as green may be a completely repulsive color. Dislike of green is not the same as being unable to see green and being ignorant of what is meant by the word "green" when it is used in conversation, as happens with colorblind people.

In any language the spoken or written name of a color triggers an image of the same color in your mind, although it may be a bit lighter or darker than what is seen in another's mind. And even that can be adjusted with additional information.

The word "red" means red to everyone who can see red, and "yellow" brings to mind yellow and not black. We rely on the constancy of our color vocabulary to assure us that traffic will stop when a traffic light is red so that we will be safe crossing the street. We rely on it when we look for signs of green spots on bread to check if the bread is moldy. We rely on red and yellow lights to let us know when electric appliances are on. We rely on color cues to help us recognize people, places, and objects from a distance.

In some cultures, people are attuned to more variations in a given color, simply because those variations are so important to survival. Those who live in the Arctic regions have many names for variations of white and few names for other colors. Those whose live in the African bush have developed many names for variations of green and for shadows. This is perfectly understandable. Those colors are important to them in their daily lives. The delicate variations have special significance for them.

COLORS AND FEELINGS

Languages are also full of figurative use of color. Color names are used to represent moods, thoughts, and feelings, partly because colors can actually trigger such feelings. Humans everywhere are similarly affected by similar colors. We can easily guess what people mean when they say they are "blue." The color blue, even if you are not feeling blue, is a subdued one; it has a calming or "toning-down" effect. We also know what it means when someone has a "red hot" feeling. Haven't we all seen fire and felt its heat? Do any more such clichés come to mind? Now, you need not get white as a ghost! No, I hope you stay in the pink and read on.

Colors are such an important part of human communication, that some cultures have assigned them mystical meanings and powers. But we do not intend to deal with that here, and add to the existing confusion about colors. Colors are known, however, to have a real physical effect on people. It has been proven that the color red, for instance, can trigger the speeding up of heart beats. It attracts attention quickly and works with adrenalin to quicken your heart beat and send you into action. This has led many to associate red with love, because love is said to do the same thing to the heart. Those who wish that a mate's heart would flutter for them may try to speed up the process with a red box of candy or some other red token of affection. Red has also been chosen as the color of danger for the very same reason.

COLORS IN NATURE

In nature, it is often yellow rather than red that signals danger. Poisonous snakes and poisonous plants are frequently yellow. Most living creatures do not see colors, or at least they do not see all the colors we can see, but yellow must be one of the colors they see clearly. Fish and bugs can see more in the ultraviolet spectrum—a light that we humans cannot see without instruments. But cats, who have keen night vision, have poor color vision. Butterflies are attracted by yellow and blue, and gardeners will tell you that slugs favor the color green.

And, contrary to popular opinion, bulls cannot see the color red. The audience at the bullfight is excited by the red that is fluttered about with great flourish. (Remember the adrenalin reaction we discussed earlier?) The bulls are attracted mainly to the movements of the man and the cloth. How do we know this? Because no matter what color cloth is flung before them, bulls react the same way while audiences respond more to the color red, which also reminds them of blood.

Some of the early and still unrefuted research in animal vision was done at the turn of the 20th century by Mrs. Christine Ladd-Franklin, a professor of psychology at Johns Hopkins University, who published her theory on color vision in 1892 following research in the lab of Dr. Hermann von Helmholtz in Berlin. (Like Madame Marie Curie, Mrs. Ladd-Franklin did not hold a doctorate for many years because women were not allowed to be registered in such programs, they could only learn as assistants to masters in their field.) Mrs. Ladd-Franklin's observations have withstood the test of time. She suggested that flowers of long ago were only white, yellow, or blue. The other colors were supposedly bred by humans, rather than evolving as a natural response to the needs of birds and bees.

Only humans, it seems, see colors simply to enjoy the beauty of them. For other animals, any specialized capacities of color sight fulfill a basic necessity, permitting hunting, self protection, mating—in a word, survival. Only humans have created colors that do not appear in nature, simply for their own sake and for entertainment. Some cultures have gone out of their way to develop colors, learning which local plants or fruits would offer a stain of a certain color, combining substances that could only be mined from the earth. A great deal of money, effort, and time have been invested in making colors for use in textiles, jewelery, and furnishings. Only humans have harnessed colors for tasks that have nothing to do with basic biological needs. People have even been willing to pay fantastic sums for dyes, and to fight for control of the areas where dyes are found.

In truth, human beings—every moment of their lives—rely on color vision and color imagery to remember details, to make decisions, to judge differences, to react to situations, to ward off danger, and to communicate information as well as to enhance the atmosphere in which they live. Yet most people don't really know what "color" is.

WHAT ARE COLORS?

Colors are "something out there" that are a way to describe things. It could be said that colors are fractured light beams. But the notion of colors simply being lights is not enough to explain what colors are. To say that colors are created when light bounces off dyes or pigments of one sort or another is not altogether correct either. We see the colors of rainbows and soap bubbles even though there are no pigments and no dyes involved.

Nor are the colors of rainbows and soap bubbles due to any reflections of anything nearby. To say that surface tensions of raindrops or soap bubbles caused light beams to bounce in such a way that our eyes recorded a color also leaves us with a limited explanation.

Furthermore, the exact mechanism by which the eye receives what the mind perceives to be color is still a puzzle to be solved. Because of the complexity of the problem, researchers will be looking with wonder at the eye and the whole visual system for a long time to come. One of the questions with which scientists are grappling deals with the mind's role in perceiving and responding to colors. It is known that we react to certain colors so consistently that advertisers know that they can anticipate certain reactions to certain colors. But there are people who do not see colors and some who confuse the colors they do see. It is known that these conditions can be inherited, and the colors that are likely to be confused are also known. Scientists know, too, which colors can disappear from our vision if we have certain illnesses. Considering the importance of color in our lives, loss of color vision can be quite distressing.

THE HUMAN FACTOR

People can manage with limited color vision, they can even manage without any color vision. But lack of color vision can make life rather dull. And confusing colors—either consistently or only under certain light conditions—can be quite annoying and depressing. It may cause others to think we are either fools or jokers.

In some instances, people do not realize that they see colors differently than others do until some event, a "failure" of some sort, enters their lives. A student may fail to follow directions in school because he confused a color that was mentioned in the instructions, or he may be unable to figure out colors in a geography or chemistry class. He or she may put away the red toy truck instead of the black one or be laughed at for filling in a face with the color green. A person may have trouble figuring out traffic lights and when to cross the street. Or an individual may first discover this condition later in life when he or she fails to see which electrical wire matches another, annoys his or her mate because socks never match, or loses his dream to fly planes when he is told he will never become a pilot.

For those who have had many such failures without explanation (and there are many such people), colorblindness has been more than a baffling stumbling block; it has often been a reason to feel like a social outcast. These people often feel as though they are being punished for something they did not cause—something they do not understand and cannot fight or correct. The very fact that so few of these people have spoken up is part of the reason the problem has been neglected for so long.

Considering that the use of colors as codes for information has increased significantly in recent years, constant color vision confusion can cause significant problems. Yet computer programmers, educators, guidance counselors, and the general public remain unconcerned—even unaware—of the problems associated with limited color vision.

It may be very soothing for those with color confusion to know that others have it, too. And it will be very useful for those who produce visual information to give more attention to this rather large group of consumers. The rest of us ought to admit that a group that makes up nearly 10 percent of the world's population deserves more understanding, not jeering laughter. Colorblindness is no joke.

Actually, I prefer to call the condition "color vision confusion" or CVC for short, for this is what it really is. I will sometimes use the word colorblindness in this book, because it is the term most commonly used, but please be aware that this same expression is sometimes used by others to mean "fairness to racial groups." It is not my intent to confuse. After all, this book is meant to present a clear picture of a real and long-ignored problem. So let's get started.

1

Vision and Perception

The mystery of how and why we see, and the extent to which we are affected by what we see have been haunting people since ancient times. Although the mystery has yet to be completely unraveled, there are many things we know about the mechanics of vision. In order to help us understand color vision and some of the problems associated with it, let's begin by looking at what we know about sight.

THE MECHANICS OF VISION

We have all heard that the eye is like a camera. Both have windows through which light enters, and both control the amount of light coming in, to prevent damage through overexposure and to admit maximum light in dim conditions. In the human eye, light travels through the clear, curved cornea which bends the light so that it can pass through the opening in the iris called the pupil. Light then passes through the lens, which focuses the light onto the retina. The retina converts light rays into electro-chemical messages or nerve impulses and sends these impulses along the optic nerve to the brain.

The Retina

Sight itself begins with the retina, a complex network of interconnective nerve cells. No one has yet untangled them, but it is known that five different types of nerve cells can be found in the retina. Beginning at the very back of the retina are the first type of nerve cells—light-sensitive or photoreceptor cells called rods and cones. Next, moving from back to front, are the horizontal cells, the bipolar cells, the amacrine cells, and the ganglion cells.

The center of the retina is the *macula*. The center of the macula is the *fovea*. The exact center of the macula is also known as the *fovea centralis*. This is the source of the sharpest image. Its position determines the place where light is brought into the sharpest focus. The fovea is responsible for detail and color discrimination, particularly the color green. It is the location of the highest concentration of cones. When you look at something directly in front of you, the image falls on the fovea where vision is well detailed, sensitive to movement, and in color. This direct sight, in contrast to peripheral vision, is the clearest path of sight, unhindered by photoreceptors or any other filters. The brain receives most of its visual information from the fovea by way of the optic nerve.

The retina can absorb, construct, expand the view, and focus on details with amazing speed. It functions effectively even while adjusting to varied light sources and clarity. The retina goes beyond what a camera can do, and does so at a flash. Exactly how this is done, no one knows as yet, but the retina's abilities rest in large part with the cells called rods and cones.

Rods and Cones

More than 130 million specialized cells in the retina act as vision receptors. These cells are called rods and cones because they actually have these shapes when viewed with a microscope. The rods distinguish black from white and are sensitive enough to work even in dim light. There are many types of cones, each type is sensitive to different types of lightwaves. The cones that are more sensitive to long wavelengths translate reds; the cones that are more sensitive to medium wavelengths translate greens; and the cones that are more sensitive to short wavelengths translate blues. When both cones and rods work properly, the cones supply the information about colors or hues, and the rods supply information about light or intensity or chroma (the strength or brightness of a color) to the brain.

These specialized cells in the eye are made of a protein called *opsin*. Opsin needs to be well nourished, particularly with vitamin A. Vitamin A is not produced by the body and, therefore, must be consumed regularly. Among the foods that contain vitamin A are green-leafed vegetables like collards and turnip greens, as well as fruits and vegetables that have the coloration of sweet potatoes, apricots, and carrots. (In fact, vitamin A was once referred to as "carotin.")

Vitamin A is needed because it contains a fat-soluble compound that is needed for the development and repair of cones and rods. But people who have color vision confusion of one sort or another are not necessarily lacking vitamin A. If they are completely colorblind, they either have no cones, or dysfunctional ones. People who are partially colorblind either lack one or more type of cones, or the cones that they do have are dysfunctional.

The cones help us have color vision while the rods deal with adjusting to light and dark. If any rods or cones are missing or functioning poorly, a problem in visual communication occurs.

Cones

Some say that cones record colors. Actually, they don't really do that. They seem to translate various lightwaves into specific electro-chemical signals that stimulate the brain to construct an image. In plain language, cones translate colors for the brain. It has been determined that there are specific wavelengths of light that are needed to see colors. (see Table 1 for the wavelengths of colors.)

Table 1   Colors in the Light Spectrum

Color	Wavelength in Nanometers
Violet	400-440
Blue	440-500
Green	500-570
Yellow	570-590
Orange	590-610
Red	610-700

We can see colors because of the unequal stimulation of the different types of cones. We can see white when all types of cones are stimulated approximately equally. Each rod or cone contains what is called a "visual pigment" that absorbs some wavelengths better than others. Rods, responsible for the ability to see in dim light, have pigment with a peak sensitivity at about 510 nanometers, in the green part of the spectrum as seen in Table 1. The pigments in the cones have peak absorptions at about 450, 530, and 560 nanometers.

Remember, each type of cone responds better to wavelengths in a certain range, but not exclusively to those wavelengths.

In order for the eye to catch the wavelength of light that will register as a color, cones must work properly. In addition, the proper number of cones must be in place. This is somewhat like having many television channels available. You can see certain channels only if you are hooked into cable service. This cable service offers you boosted signals. What's more, a television set that receives these signals must be plugged in and must be operational in order for you to receive the signals. Furthermore, if the television is not set to translate the waves into color messages—if, for instance, it is a black and white television set—no color will be seen even if the signals have been received. All of the factors must be in place for the full picture to emerge with all the details.

Rods
Rods are elongated tube-shaped cells with light-sensitive tips. They stand packed like blades of grass on a golf course and are rooted in the membrane of the retina. While cones are concentrated in the fovea, the rest of the retina contains primarily rods.

The rods offer information about light and shading. Shading is an important bit of information. It can help us to determine depth or roundness and inform us of whether something is wet or dry. Shading can help us to judge what time of day it is, what the environmental conditions are like, and much more. We know that rods do not play a significant role in color vision, because our ability to see colors is very limited in dim light. Just look around you on a dark night. Most things appear to you in shades of gray.

About 120 million rods per eye are needed for the proper balance of peripheral and night vision. Rods are roughly 100 times more sensitive to light than cones. Each rod contains millions of molecules of rhodopsin, a chemical that is very sensitive to light. If rods are missing or damaged for any reason, night blindness and visual impairment will occur, particularly limitation of shades.

WHAT IS COLOR?

It may be said that colors are fractured light beams. But the notion of colors simply being lights is not enough to explain what colors are. To say that colors are created when light bounces off dyes or pigments of one sort or another is not altogether correct either because we see the colors of rainbows and soap bubbles although there are no pigments and no dyes involved. Nor are the colors of rainbows and soap bubbles due to any reflections of anything near them. To say that surface tensions of raindrops or soap bubbles cause light beams to bounce in such a way that our eyes record a color also leaves us with a limited explanation of what we have seen. In fact, colors and light beams are as elusive as they have ever been, but it has been determined that certain wavelengths of light permit us to see certain colors (as shown in Table 1, page 9).

Color can be spoken of in terms of the observer or of the light. When we talk about the color of objects or chroma—as the observer sees it—we speak of hue, chroma, and saturation. Because color can be considered both a function of light and a function of an observer, color can be spoken of in physiological and psychological terms as well.

In a purely physiological or biological sense, color is the consequence of unequal stimulation of a number of cones. A green leaf, for instance, absorbs long and short wavelength light and reflects light of middle wavelengths. But it is not only the eyes that are involved in seeing colors. Our brains have a part to play, too. Our brains make sense of the information that is transmitted by the eyes. What's more, we may not make note of certain details that our eyes register unless our brains signal that the detail is important. Detecting color depends on the functioning of the light-sensitive cells in the retina and on the brain's interpretation of the information received from the eye. Because of the brain's role, psychologists have long studied color vision as a developmental process.

THE DEVELOPMENT OF COLOR VISION IN HUMANS

Have you ever seen colored objects hung above a crib or carriage to entertain an infant? Of course! But there is no proof that children can see colors distinctly at an early age. We know that it takes many weeks before they actually see anything clearly at all. Color vision may or may not develop at the same rate.

At the turn of the century, a developmental psychologist named James Mark Baldwin conducted a test on his own infant daughter. The test showed that she clearly responded to colored items more than to those lacking color. Subsequent research has supported

Baldwin's conclusions that children do register colors at an early age.

As children grow, their need for color names grows. Colors become adjectives, tools for being more descriptive in verbal communication. Colors can be a means of expressing feelings or preferences. By kindergarten age, children are expected to learn which color is which and to respond when asked about colors. They are asked to color pictures as they learn the basics of nursery rhymes, and they are asked to match geometric shapes which are, these days, colored.

By this time, children differentiate colors, and they also can make sense of variations of shading of colors. But it is difficult to pin down the extent to which the child will give a "real" response or a "make believe" response. Color vision problems, therefore, are often not diagnosed in very young children.

It is, of course, possible to diagnose nearsightedness or farsightedness. Such vision can be tested with the aid of an instrument called an autoreferactor, but color vision confusion cannot be detected in this manner. At the kindergarten level, children are at their imaginative prime, going in and out of flights of fancy. They often "color" their answers.

Responses of children aged seven and up are more dependable. By that age, children can be tested more reliably. Sadly, they rarely are tested for color vision confusion. Color vision has not been considered a matter of serious importance. There are art therapy textbooks that do not even mention the possibility that children might be colorblind.

Color vision confusion leads to various problems. If a parent or teacher is attuned to the problem, it can be better dealt with. I wish to stress that colors are not just a willy nilly way of expressing yourself in an art classroom. If a child constantly confuses colors, it may not be stupidity, it may well be colorblindness. In Chapter Two, we will learn exactly what the condition is.

2

What Is
Colorblindness?

"I just don't see it!" Have you ever heard anyone say this? Maybe you have said it yourself. Does it mean you are stupid? Does it mean that you do not grasp information? Does it mean you are blind?

No, it usually means that some aspect of the larger sum of information is unclear to you, no matter how hard you try to focus on it. This is not unlike what the colorblind person experiences, except that for such a person, some aspect of the sum total will forever remain unclear.

Colorblindness is a problem in seeing colors as most others see them. But colorblind people are not blind. They usually have keen eyesight, and if they do not, their visual impairment has nothing to do with their colorblindness. Colorblind people tend to confuse some colors and may not see other colors at all. Cases differ. Some seem to see all colors when shown one at a time, but then find it hard to decipher colors that are mingled. Some may be unable to match some colors in certain lights. Only a rare few do not see colors at all. According to official figures, more than 8 percent of the male population in America has color vision confusion. In addition, it is estimated that 2 percent of women—yes, women—have this problem. I estimate that the number is much higher for both sexes.

It is hard to say exactly how many people have color vision confusion because no extensive studies have been done on the subject. Many people who are colorblind have been reluctant to speak about it, and few others have taken the condition seriously. Because of this "blindness" to color vision confusion, no studies have been done with large groups of cooperative colorblind people.

The existing statistics are the results of limited testing. Who was tested? People who attempted to get certain jobs, people who wanted to join the navy or air force, and a few others, but for most jobs, there is no testing for color vision. There has been no nationwide testing in schools, and no testing of adults when they apply for driver's licenses.

Statistics for women are particularly sketchy. Why? For the most part, until recent years, women have had a hard time getting into those fields that require tests for color vision. Women were not hired as airline pilots, ship's captains, railroad engineers, electrical contractors, or managers of pharmaceutical plants. Nor were they drafted into the military. The screening of applicants for these jobs has supplied most of the statistics regarding color vision confusion among men. (You can read more about CVC and women in Chapter 6.)

Now, if you consider that the total population of the United States is somewhere around 280 million, and about half of these people are males, at least 140 million Americans are males. And 8 percent of that— 11 million—is not a small number. Those 11 million colorblind men often have not voiced their condition because they hardly pay any attention to colors. Colors have not been the subject of masculine conversation, nor have most jobs like mechanic, farmer, insurance salesman, engineer, or accountant been considered to require color vision. Colorblind men have tended to find spouses who are understanding and who can cover for the condition, choosing clothes and other things of color for them. Their problems have been hidden in other ways, as they tend to pick hobbies and recreational activities that do not require acute color vision but that will allow them to express their creativity. Such people are not usually included in any statistics.

To get a more accurate picture of the number of people who have CVC, we must figure in the undiscovered men as well as the females who are colorblind. We also have to add the untold numbers who acquire the condition at some point in their lives.

INHERITED COLORBLINDNESS

Most colorblind people are born with this problem. It is probably caused by genes inherited through the mother, although she may not show any signs of it herself. A woman can exhibit colorblindness if she inherits genes that are faulty from both her mother and her father.

Genes that deal with color vision were discovered some years ago on the long arm of the X chromosome, which is carried doubly by females. More than fifty years ago, George Waaler, a Danish physiologist, discovered that colorblindness is a condition in which a defective gene is inherited from the mother. In 1986, the location of the defective genes responsible for the inheritance of color vision confusion was identified by Dr. Jeremy Nathans. His discovery was made when he was assistant professor of molecular biology and genetics at the Howard Hughes Medical Institute of Johns Hopkins University School of Medicine.

But once the location of the genes was discovered, additional research led to other startling findings. The husband and wife team of Jay and Maureen Neitz, researchers in different departments of the University of Wisconsin Medical College—one a geneticist working with the Department of Opthalmology and the other working with the Department of Cellular Biology and Anatomy focusing on the mechanics of sight—put their findings together and concluded in 1994 that:

- People who have full color vision have not one, but as many as ten color vision genes, and people who are colorblind have as many genes as those with full color vision.

- Not all the color vision genes seem to be of equal strength; some may be more powerful than others. As a result, the more powerful genes may drown out the rods and cones that are produced by the weaker genes.

- All of the common color vision deficiencies can be explained by a mutation of the genes that produce the pigments required for normal color vision, and the inability to see some colors may be due to lack of genes.

In short, the Neitz researchers found that some people have more colorvision genes—as many as ten in some people—with each gene affecting a degree of light vision and the ability to see as many as two colors. These colors are not simply red or blue or green, but variations such as violet and other colors, and these genes may interchange locations with others, leading to some confusing results.

This finding opened the door to fresh considerations as to why people have varied levels of color vision confusion—why some have it more in one eye than in another, why some see colors far less distinctly under certain conditions—and other questions about the mechanics and genetics of color vision confusion.

But what was most startling to Jay and Maureen Neitz was that their discovery seemed to negate the long-held Young-Helmholz Theory. The Young-Helmholz Theory held that there was just one gene that enabled us to see all colors through the mixing of blue, green, and red light-waves. The Neitz Theory posited the existence of many genes responsible for a variety of colors and shades. This discovery will doubtlessly lead to greater and clearer understanding of the causes of color vision disturbances for those who have inherited colorblindness.

A recent study in China suggests it may soon be possible to determine if a child is colorblind at birth by studying the loops in the design of the fingerprints. It has even been suggested that by getting information about infants' tendencies toward color vision problems, we can determine if a child is genetically predisposed to one of the ailments that cause color vision loss later in life.

It appears, for instance, that the gene that is important for the maintenance of red blood cell glucose metabolism is also located on the long arm of the X chromosome. This gene, if defective, can lead to the development of diabetes (an imbalance in the absorption of glucose by the blood) and colorblindness. Sickle cell anemia is another inherited blood ailment that leads to color vision loss as it progresses. The relationship of inherited diseases to color vision loss has only become apparent in recent years. This is partly because many people with inherited conditions first start exhibiting colorblindness during their adult years, and only recently have so many people with inherited chronic ailments managed to live to adulthood. Furthermore, records regarding the onset of colorblindness late in life are scant. In many instances, doctors have not considered color vision a significant issue and haven't tested for, or even inquired about it.

ACQUIRED COLORBLINDNESS

Adults who have no genetic problems linked to color vision confusion can also acquire this condition. Loss of color vision can be acquired as a result of illnesses such as multiple sclerosis or as a result of taking certain medications. In addition, more and more environmental factors such as industrial pollution have been linked to colorblindness, and the sun is another culprit. (See Chapter 5, Causes of Color Vision Confusion, for more information on medications and environmental factors leading to CVC.)

Acquired color vision defects tend to be progressive in nature, getting worse with time. If, however, the source of the problem is removed, the condition gets better with time. Of course, people who have color vision loss because of chronic ailments that worsen over time can do little about it. People who take certain medications that are crucial for a stable life will have to put up with this side effect. Hopefully, as the problem of color vision confusion becomes better understood, researchers will look for drugs that do not have this side effect.

IN SCIENTIFIC TERMS

Most colorblind people have inherited the condition. They inherit genes that cause them to develop faulty rods or cones, or both. Or else, they have an insufficient number of rods or cones to be properly effective for complete color sight. It may also be that they cannot produce the right amount of opsin, the protein that is the basis of the cones and rods, that is needed to create and keep them in good repair.

In some instances, the gene for color vision may be fine, but the gene that tells the chemicals that trigger the color vision gene to function may be defective. These chemicals are called enzymes. Cells all over the body are moved to action as the result of enzymes that are specially designed to tell them to go to work. Even these enzymes have inherited information about how to behave.

Genes, microscopic message carriers in the cells of our bodies, are inherited from our mothers and fathers. We inherit eye color, hair color, even the length of fingers from our parents. Each bit of information pertaining to development of any inherited characteristic is transferred from the parent to the child through a gene. These genes came to us when our mother's and father's sex cells joined to develop the first cell that made up our bodies.

Genes are a significant part of the package created when the mother's egg, or ovum, and the father's sperm join to create the new life form, the new cell that grows to become a new human being. But the genes do not transfer one by one. They transfer in groups of genes located within structures called chromosomes. Each human cell has 46 chromosomes, with the exception of ovum in females, and sperm in males—these only have 23 chromosomes. The chromosomes that determine an individual's sex are paired into either two X's (XX) in females, or an X and a Y (XY) in males. However, the sex cells (ovum and sperm) are not paired. The ova has a lone X, and the sperm has an X or a Y. These lone chromosomes carry only half of the genetic information from the carrier. The reason is simple. If they contained a full complement of forty-six chromosomes, they would not be able to join with another cell to make up the "whole" number. A fertilized egg automatically receives an X from the mother, and either an X or a Y from the father. When an egg is fertilized by a sperm, the offspring receives the combined genetic information from the chromosomes of each parent.

Imagine the possible variations of features that can be inherited! But once the union has taken place, the combination that wins out is the one that is in charge of the new cell.

Why Does This Matter?

This explains to us how it is that a boy inherits colorblindness from his mother. The genes that are responsible for color vision are on the X chromosome, and if these genes are faulty, the boy will have color vision confusion. As we pointed out before, a girl inherits one X chromosome from her mother and one from her father, whereas a boy has only one, which he inherited from his mother. A girl who has one X chromosome with a faulty gene will have normal color vision as long as the gene on her other X chromosome is normal (she will, however, be a "carrier"). She will be colorblind only if she has inherited two faulty X chromosomes—one from her mother and one from her father. But a boy will be colorblind from birth with only the one X chromosome carrying a faulty gene.

The genes that carry the basic inherited information regarding color vision are passed on by the mother. In other words, if a father is colorblind, that will not cause his son to be colorblind. His genes for color vision alone will not affect his son.

If a woman carries the genes for colorblindness, her son will be colorblind if he inherits the faulty X that she carries. She may not show any signs of color vision confusion or even know about it. But she can transfer these genes to her son. The mother may be carrying a gene she inherited from a colorblind father or mother—or from a mother whose own vision was normal, but who carried a faulty color vision gene—and she can transfer it to her son. (There are several different types of inherited and acquired color vision confusion that are discussed in the next chapter.)

IN HUMAN TERMS

A colorblind person can hardly explain the condition to others. Even if colorblind people do explain, few people really believe or understand what they are told.

The colors seen by colorblind people are not the colors you and I expect them to see. For this reason, their vocabulary of colors is not the same as the vocabulary of those with full color vision. What's more, colorblind people often have to figure out what others expect them to see. After all, these people do not act as if they are in any way visually handicapped, nor do they seem confused or incapable of understanding information. Others, therefore, make no concessions when dealing with the colorblind and often mistake the responses they get for silliness or stupidity. I assure you that colorblind people are not acting as they do in order to gain attention. And yet, many people who have the problem have been accused of just that.

"If you would only pay attention and make an effort," so many colorblind people have been told at one time or another in their lives, "you could learn color names." But it isn't that they do not know color names or that they do not register them in their minds. It isn't that they are not paying attention. They simply do not see the colors that others see, but they are very attuned to differentiations in variations of tones—the variation of lightness or darkness—of colors they do see, and they tend to notice things that those who see colors often ignore.

IN SUMMARY

At some time or another, we all mix up some visual information. The sunlight might have been too strong or the indoor lighting might have been too weak. Our eyes might have been tired or watery. For most, this is simply a transitory happening, something that passes within moments.

But for some people, this condition, this mixing up of colors, or this inability to notice some of them altogether, is a long-term or permanent factor. They cannot rely on the colors they see to give them information or to be a clue to bits of information they needed to remember. Making mistakes about visual information can be confusing and costly. Missing visual information can be as much of a problem as missing words in spoken sentences. It can be very frustrating both to the person who aims to communicate the information and the person who needs to act on the information.

Miscommunication may be lessened if you remember the following:

- Colorblindness is not a form of blindness.
- You cannot catch colorblindness from anyone around you.
- You cannot cure colorblindness with medication, operations, or diet.
- You can inherit or acquire colorblindness.
- Most people who have this condition see some colors. A rare few see no colors.

If you are colorblind, remember that you are not alone. If your problem is due to inherited tendencies, there is, as yet, no relief. But there are compensatory and coping skills you can learn. Someday—maybe sooner than you think—gene therapy may be available. Gene therapy is now being developed for all sorts of purposes. Missing genes have been added and genes have been altered. In some cases, defective genes have been discarded.

If your colorblindness was acquired, you may find that you have choices to make. The decisions may not be easy. Knowing how to effectively deal with colorblindness may make the choices easier.

3

Types of Colorblindness

Once upon a time, people who could not see any or all of various colors were called Daltonics because a British scientist named John Dalton was the first to write about this condition. In Spain and France, the condition is still referred to as Daltonism or Dalton Mania. In today's scientific jargon, people who have full color vision are called trichromats. Those who can see only two of the three primary colors of light (red, green, and blue, as opposed to red, yellow, and blue, which are primary colors in paint) are referred to as dichromats. A very small number of people have achromatopsia, the inability to see any colors.

So far, we've looked at the causes and manifestations of color vision confusion in general. Let's now look at the specific colors and that present problems. We'll examine each form of CVC in some detail and discuss some of the ways confusing these colors can interfere with daily life.

DICHROMATISM

Among those who inherit color vision confusion there are three basic groups that we will discuss here.

Deuteranopia

Those who have this form of color vision confusion have difficulty when dealing with green. They make up one of the largest groups of colorblind people. Very often they also have a problem with red.

People who have this condition may recognize any color if they can contrast the color in question with another color in good light. They can often see red or green if the item that is red or green is held against another color. In other words, if their eyes can compare colors, they seem to be able to distinguish red and green. They will be able to pick out red or green from a pack of colored papers, but if you hand them something that is red or green and ask them what color they see, they will be a bit puzzled. It seems as though they have a red-green "weakness." At 500 nanometers deuteronopians and protanopians see a colorless white.

Protanopia

People who have this form of CVC often seem to need an abnormal amount of red or have no sense of red colorvision. Most often, people with this condition see bold red as black or as nonexistent. Many in this group react to red or green only when the colors "scream." Chances are, these people do not actually see red or green even then, but are simply sensing some color.

Such people may see red-orange as brown and yellow-green as brown. In other words, neither red nor green provides sure visual information. Neither color can be seen or recorded properly by the eye. For this reason, people with this condition may say that red and green are the same, or they have a mental image of two different browns.

Tritanopia

Those who have problems distinguishing blue and/or yellow are blue-yellow colorblind. This disorder is much less common than red-green colorblindness, and is most often acquired, not inherited. These people may see both blue and yellow as white. They may even see mint green or pink as an equal to light blue.

RED COLOR VISION CONFUSION

Red color vision confusion is the most common type of inherited colorblindness. Some people with this disorder do not have the cones needed to see red. This means that they do not see red at all, or they see it as black. Others have defective red cones, and that leads them to see red as equal to dark brown or orange.

RED'S ODD HISTORY

Red has been very expensive to produce throughout history, and therefore, used very sparingly. The first cheap commercially available red was alizarin crimson, developed in the mid 1800s by the British chemist William Henry Perkins, while doing research at a German dye laboratory. It was made from an extract of a plant called "madder" that was grown extensively in Turkey. Germany thus had the patent on commercial red dye. Following the First World War, Britain boycotted products from Germany, leading some to make fortunes in smuggling red dye from Germany to Britain due to industrial demands.

There has also been some controversy in this country over a food coloring agent known as red dye number 2, which was used mostly in candy. Studies conducted in Russia in 1970 revealed that this dye could possibly be a cancer-causing agent, so it was banned in the United States in 1976. Many candy companies stopped producing red candy altogether for a while, because the consumers still considered it "taboo." (Because the studies could not prove that the dye was a carcinogen, Canada still uses this dye in foods and candy.)

People who have this form of CVC often also have difficulty differentiating orange, yellow, and green. Those who have a problem with both green and red may tell you that green is red or red is green because both appear the same to them. It may also be that they mistake both red and green for either orange or brown.

They do seem to see blue although they may include purple as blue. It is the red component in purple that makes it look different from blue to people with full color vision. These people may also see orange as yellow for the same reason; orange is yellow with a bit of red in it. Some may also see yellow as green.

Some Daily Problems and Adjustments

For people who have red or green CVC, driving at night can be a real problem. Heading to shore with a boat after sundown can similarly be a problem, if you cannot see visual cues like traffic lights, tail lights, or buoy lights. Red and green are the lights that inform a boater or driver whether it is safe to head forward or whether it is necessary to take steps to avoid an accident. Red, when seen as black or dark brown against the blackness of a night sky, seems to disappear alto-gether. If a signal is only a red blinker on a country crossroad, you can imagine what a problem it is; the blinker doesn't give any warning at all. There have been many times when a red traffic or warning light was not obeyed, not because it was ignored, but because it was truly not seen. If, after an accident, one of the drivers involved says he never saw the light, he may be telling the truth. Furthermore, when driving at night, it is more difficult for the person with red color vision confusion to check the dashboard, where details and emer-gency lights are often highlighted in red against a black background.

Docking boats at night requires following buoy instructions. Buoys are lit with red lights. Against a night sky, they too "disappear," and the docking may have to be done by guesswork. A yachtsman with red CVC may find himself on a sandbar or may damage another boat because of inability to distinguish buoy lights.

Remember the colorblind fiber optics scientist we met on page x, who deals with audio rather than visual transmission because he can't see the colors? He has a real problem driving at night because he can-not distinguish which are street lights and which are traffic lights. He does not see red at all so he cannot tell if he is passing a red light. He carefully watches the rest of the traffic to see when other motorists stop. But the system isn't foolproof; he has gotten a number of tickets for jumping lights. He does not see the red of the brake lights, but he can see brake lights that are amber. Some car makers have changed the color of the brake lights but most models still have red ones.

Some people with red color confusion have said that their spouses complain because they do not enjoy the color of a beautiful sunset, nor can they properly choose fruit and vegetables in stores. And peo-ple with this form of CVC are sometimes utterly repulsed by foods that quite often appear black or some indistinct color. Lipstick may look black. Blond hair may look green. And, of course, there is always the problem of picking clothes. Reading signs can also be a problem.

Red exit signs in a darkened auditorium are of no help to someone who has red CVC. The red registers as black and gets lost in the black-ness of the auditorium. Manny, aged 61, still shudders when he recalls the extent to which he was afraid to go to the movies when he was a child because if he had to go to the bathroom, he could not find the door. His mother had told him that the door is below the sign marked E-X-I-T, but he never saw such a sign. In those days, the signs were lit in red. In many places, they still are, but some establishments have recently begun to use green signs. Green exit signs in a darkened auditorium can be seen by everybody, including those who have green color vision confusion. Those with green colorblindness will see the signs as white, which can easily be read against the darkened auditorium walls.

Red CVC can also affect people's careers. Sometimes, we hear of "cold-blooded" surgeons. These doctors may not really be cold blooded, but blood may appear less repulsive to them than it does to most of us. If they have red CVC, they may see blood as dark brown or black. These colors may not be as upsetting to look at as bright red, so their reaction to blood may be different.

As early as 1881, it was noted that doctors involved with surgery may often be red color-deficient. At that time in the United States, a Dr. D.S. White noted that a significant number of surgeons had trouble when looking through ophthalmoscopes because they could not distinguish red blood vessels. It was suggested that the color confusion might be a blessing in disguise for these doctors, enabling them to become surgeons while other very bright medical students did not.

In other fields, red CVC is less of a boon. Consider those who work with electrical equipment. Electrical machinery that has a red on-off light or digital numbers in red on a black background can become a hazard. If you do not know whether a tool is off or on, or if you cannot read information that appears on gauges, dangerous problems can occur.

Color vision confusion can be troublesome for businessmen in some unusual ways. Take the travelling salesman who told me how stunned he was to learn that the car he had owned for almost three years was not red but orange. To make matters worse for this very conservative gentleman, it was a rather rude hue of orange at that. The color had apparently cost him some business deals as well as a wife who got fed up—she hated his selection of "red." When he finished relating his story, this businessman turned to me and said, "Is my face red? I wouldn't know."

GREEN COLOR VISION CONFUSION

Although green color vision confusion is caused by faulty or missing cones, green is the color to which rods are most sensitive. If the cones

---

GREEN'S ODD HISTORY

For a long time, the color green was excluded from industry when it was at all possible. Not only did green represent bile and greed, but poison, too. For instance, the paint color Paris green, which is similar to emerald green, was taken off the market in 1878 after it was shown that it caused poisoning of children who had toys painted with it. A green dye produced with arsenic had been used in the textile industry until it was shown that people who wore articles of clothing made with this dye could be poisoned by it. Workers who handled the dye were also in danger. Sheele's green, which was manufactured by the Sheele Company in Germany a century ago, was also proven to be poisonous when used as a tint in the cream that garnishes cakes.

---

and rods are seriously defective, people may say that green is yellow, blue, grey, white, or even orange. They will also see yellow as a "reddish" color or orange. It is common for them to confuse red and green.

While the worst case scenario for those with red color vision loss is to see red as black, those who have the worst case of green cone malfunction see green as white. This whiteness can, in turn, affect the rods, which have to adjust to the excess light of the white. (You will recall that rods play a role in adjusting light and dark vision and the relativity of shades.)

Someone who has red CVC may not see the crowns of tulips in a field. But try to imagine sitting at a baseball game and seeing the field as orange! Consider that if a person looks at green and says it's orange, chances are this person has no concept of what you sense when you see or even think of the color orange. It's better not to try to understand the problem from your perspective, but to accept that this person has another visual system and may even express delight at the sight of the "orange" field, although if he saw an orange span of color he might say it is red, or green. He may even love green or white hair, which may be, in fact, blonde.

Some Daily Problems and Adjustments

For those who have green CVC, the color green, particularly in daytime, may be seen as a grey, white, or yellow. Drivers with green CVC have reported that at night, the round green traffic light looks no different than the street lights to them. For these people, green traffic lights are confused with other lights and are, therefore, not useful cues.

A North Carolina boy with green CVC was nearly thrown out of school for being totally uncooperative. He was repeatedly punished by his teacher because he constantly "refused" to copy what she wrote on the board. He claimed he did not see anything on the board although he did see her writing on it. It took a great deal of time and effort to convince school authorities that the boy wasn't being disobedient. He simply could not read what was written with yellow chalk on a green board. To him, the colors looked the same—white.

His parents had no idea that he could not see green. But they knew he was not a defiant child, and they managed to find the reason for their son's odd behavior. The boy was allowed to stay in school only after his parents brought in an expert to prove he had green color vision confusion.

The ability to differentiate green is also important in many vocational fields. How, for instance, does one optician with green confusion deal with sunglasses? He tints glasses "by the numbers." He chooses the shade of green from numbered samples rather than by matching the colors. The optician found a solution to his problem, but others are still working on it. Peter Seibel, a prominent investigator of maritime accidents, is quite vocal about recognizing the serious problems that green color vision confusion can cause in the maritime industry.

Peter had fallen in love with boats as a child but was told he could never aspire to be a ship's captain because he is colorblind. He had known about his CVC since his kindergarten days in the 1930s when his aunt, who was his teacher, decided to test him using the newly developed Ishihara Test. Because of his aunt's understanding, Peter was never told he was stupid or blind; he was simply told he would do well to squash some dreams and develop others. This led Peter to become a mechanical engineer, then to specialize in the mechanical aspects of ships, and to become an expert on what could go wrong; why certain accidents take place. Involved in the maritime industry for more than forty years, he often conducts investigations for the insurance companies that underwrite the transport of cargo and insure ships. For relaxation, he takes his sailboat out and catches the breeze on Long Island Sound.

Peter was one of the people who was to appear in an educational video that I produced. He rushed into the studio for the taping session a little bit breathless, having just flown back from being on call at a major accident involving a Brazilian freighter. Mired with its cargo in the Savannah River, the freighter had been so mangled by the force of an impact that, according to Peter, "it looked like a bunch of metal spaghetti in there." It would take weeks to dislodge the freighter and make the proper repairs.

The cause of the accident was a lack of green color vision. You see, the captain, who had been tested for color vision, was not the one to call the orders when the ship maneuvered its way up the Savannah River. The first mate was in charge at that time, which is a common enough occurrence. Unfortunately, while a captain must pass a color vision test in order to get his license, a mate need not.

The ship had entered Savannah in the early evening. The lights of the buoys had to be followed—they are the traffic lights of the ocean. Red warns that the shipping channel is too shallow, too rocky, or poses some other hazard to a ship. Green stands for "go." The mate confused the green lights with the white lights of the properties on shore that are on private docks or denote a shoreline highway. Had the mate seen the green, he would have known that it was safe to steer the ship in the direction of the light. But because he was green color-blind, he veered off the other way to avoid an accident, straight onto a rock-filled sandbar.

One of Peter's pet peeves is that many of the chemicals used on board for the running of vessels and for cleaning and repair are colored green, or expected to be mixed with green fluids, or have to be matched against a color chart that includes green. He claims that given the large number of men who work in the maritime industry, there must be many who have green CVC. He also believes that being at sea and looking out at the glare of the sun on the water day in and day out adds to the problem.

He has often pointed out accidents that are the result of overuse, underuse, or misuse of some green chemicals and of green lights. He has asked that companies that produce the cleaners and chemicals for maritime usage change the color of the liquids. He also thinks mates as well as captains should be tested for green color vision. But for some reason, this testing has been slow in coming. Even though it has cost insurance companies, exporters, and ship owners plenty, it seems they cannot grasp that a major problem hinges on color and the color vision capacities of crews.

Gerald Murch, an electrical engineer involved with the development of computer graphics color capabilities, once told me of his personal experience with someone who has no green vision. Gerald had discovered that, by manipulations of electrical impulses, he could create colors on a computer screen. The discovery excited him so much that he ran to his boss and asked him to come see what he had created. But when his boss looked at the screen, he said, "So what!" It turned out, Gerald's boss had green CVC and saw green as white. At that time, all the information on a computer terminal appeared in white.

RED-GREEN COLOR VISION CONFUSION

Red color vision confusion is often coupled with green color vision confusion. The existence of both types of CVC has been acknowledged for more than one hundred years, since they were noted by the Scottish physicist James Clark Maxwell. People who confuse the two colors may say that green and red look alike. To them, an orange-brown or a purple-brown most closely resembles green and red. In other cases, people with red-green CVC think that a purple-brown is either red or green.

Some Daily Problems and Adjustments

Red-green CVC can be a stumbling block in simple, everyday situations. One young man confided that he had lost a number of girlfriends because he complemented them on their lovely green complexions. Of course, he should have said pink, but to him it was all the same. Then, too, while some people can decide if a pear is ripe by the yellowish coloration it has when ready to be eaten, people who have red-green color vision confusion cannot use this clue.

Red-green CVC can also present obstacles to people's careers. I know a physician's assistant who has red-green CVC. He began his career as a medic in Vietnam. Since then he has had problems checking the levels of sugar in the urine samples of diabetics. He explained that interpreting this test requires comparison of variations of greens. He got a terrible headache knowing he had to hide his problem from the patients, and had to ask the doctor's receptionist to check whether he was interpreting the color chart correctly. But he never considered what would happen if the receptionist were also colorblind! One woman who was hired as a temporary replacement was unable to help him. He thought that she was being snippy when she said she was "just a receptionist" and could not help him. Now he knows better. (Recent developments in medical technology have eliminated such problems with this test.)

This man also has trouble seeing the signs of measles, which begin as red blotches, particularly on the abdomen. He says he never had to deal with diabetes or with measles in Vietnam, and no one asked him if he was colorblind. He was known as a caring and capable medic, and his record had helped him to become a physician's assistant in civilian life.

James, a landscape architect, also has red-green confusion. To him, green is a color similar to brown. Since he also sees red as brown, green is equal to red. He still manages to do his job by focusing not on floral displays, but on the textural effects of leaves and petals and variations of tones of colors. He feels that since many architects also focus on tonality and texture, he "speaks their language." He had known of his CVC since childhood, and knew that it was not a reflection of his intelligence, although he was badgered by kids in school. He has always been aware of his color vision confusion and considers it acceptable because his grandfather had CVC, as did many of his other relatives. His colorblind uncle became a fashion designer for men. How did he manage? He has high sensitivity to details and variations of greys, weaves, and patterns. This is excellent for his needs as a conservative men's suit designer. James's cousin (his mother's sister's son), is quite successful refurbishing houses despite his CVC. He has a reputation for being careful, taking time to assure harmonious tonalities and textural combinations in his work (which some others might overlook). For this, he can command high fees.

Then there was the student who came from France and confided that he did not understand why American men wear pink pants. He was referring to the khaki-colored summer-weight pants that are so common among college students. He also explained that he does not drink wine because people expect him—a Frenchman—to be able to distinguish between white and rosé wines. To him, both look like water! Red wine looks black to him, and he doesn't particularly care for the idea of drinking a black liquid! (The aversion that develops because of the color of a beverage may explain why beer manufacturers add caramel coloring to that drink. In this way, it looks neither dark nor clear like water.)

Because the Frenchman was reluctant to admit the real reason for his not drinking wine, he invented an excuse. He said that he refrains from drinking spirits because his father is an alcoholic, but he had to admit the truth when he was "caught" drinking beer.

Incidentally, this young man was in America because he had lost his job in France and was hoping to learn another profession. In his native country, he had been a carpet repairman, a very careful craftsman with a fine grasp of the many varieties of wools. So what had happened? He had always been very reliable, so the owner of the carpet business went on vacation, leaving him in charge. One day, a long-time customer brought in a rug that he wanted repaired quickly because he was planning a party. Our repairman did a fine job—but, oh, what colors he used!

When the owner of the rug returned three days later, he was beside himself with grief and rage. He demanded that the work be undone. But our repairman was so good at delicate knots that he would have had to cut the whole area out. It was impossible. The client told others about the bad job. Thus, our repairman soon needed to find another way to make a living.

BLUE COLOR VISION CONFUSION

For some people who have this problem, pure blue wavelengths seem to "shift down," and pure green wavelengths "shift up" till the two colors appear as one. (You will recall from Chapter 1 that these two colors are very close to each other in wavelengths, so in this case they merge.) In other words, the wavelengths of both colors are perceived incorrectly, and as one color. Those who have blue color vision disturbances may also have difficulty seeing yellow; they may see it as white ranging to grey. For them, both blue and yellow become white or grey. Because green is comprised of yellow and blue, green is often confused as well. It may be called yellow or blue or grey.

Although as many females as males have blue CVC, the condition is a relatively uncommon form of color vision confusion. More often than not, it appears in people who have a physical disorder that involves more than just the cones and rods of the eyes. The condition's appearance with certain physical disorders has proven to be so reliable that blue CVC has become a clue to the existence of those physical problems. Diabetes and some liver disorders can be detected in this manner.

There are a number of males who have only a slight problem distinguishing blue; they mix it up with green. These men do not seem to have a physical disorder. It is, in fact, not uncommon for young boys to have blue/green confusion that becomes less pronounced in adulthood. It is not known whether they grow out of it or eventually develop visual cues to tell the difference.

Some Daily Problems and Adjustments

The inability to distinguish the color blue or the tendency to confuse it with white is a problem for anyone who has to follow blue lights, particularly at night. Blue CVC can be dangerous for those who cannot tell that a blue flame is on when using gas burners or welding torches. It can be a problem for anyone using chemicals in industry or cleaning solutions at home.

Many industrial chemicals are colored blue or bluish green. Often, these chemicals have to be prepared as solutions, which requires diluting them. But if you cannot see the color in the first place, it is difficult to tell whether the chemical has been appropriately mixed. Working with such chemicals can become a baffling task, indeed. And, of course, it can be a problem to select color-coordinated clothing, follow signs written in light blue, or read bills that are often printed in blue.

Blue vision confusion has kept men from becoming airplane pilots because runways are outlined with blue lights. Imagine if a pilot in flight could not distinguish a row of windows or streets and confused them with a runway because he saw them all as equal in color to white!

One of the strangest cases regarding blue CVC had to do with a person's being unable to see the flame on a gas stove. A German man who had trained to be a chef had no idea that blue vision confusion would play a role in this profession. After all, nothing we eat is blue and cakes aren't often decorated with a blue color.

This man had done well in cooking school and would have done well professionally if he had been left alone, he says. But in a restaurant kitchen, cooks have to share burners, as well as share time and space. In school, he would turn on the burner and judge the "doneness" of the food by its movement in the pot or pan. He knew which burner was turned on because he was the only one at the stove. But when he shared a stove and others turned on burners on which no pot could be placed for a given amount of time, he knew he was in trouble.

For a long time, he had no idea what was causing the skin on his right arm to flare up in an angry red rash. It began to look so bad that he was fired from different establishments. Owners did not want him handling food with such a rash. However, each time he was fired, the rash soon disappeared. This made him wonder if it was a nervous reaction, a psychosomatic rash. But on his last job, the skin of his arm became so bad, scar over scar, that he could no longer stretch the arm. The "rash" was actually caused by the burn of the blue flame that he could not see. While in rehabilitation, he took up a sport that helped develop his other arm. He became a champion Ping-Pong player and lectured at schools about choosing trades. He represented his country at the International Games for the Disabled in 1984 in the United States. (This is where I met him, as I was a volunteer German language translator.)

Blue CVC can be a significant problem to students in classes where welding is involved. A welding flame must reach a particular temperature before it can be used. Students know the temperature is right when the flame reaches a deep blue color. To compensate for their inability to see the blue, some students with blue CVC learned to focus on the white triangular design that appears at the base of the flame. The size of this triangular white area is a measure of the flame's heat, and it seems to contrast with the blue flame enough for the blue-confused eye to distinguish.

In another case, Jane, a 28-year-old woman, could not tell dark blue from black. This is a not uncommon condition. What happens is the rods seem to need far more light than normal to register dark colors. In some cases it is due to human factors such as over-exposure to light. In Jane's case, her inability to distinguish navy from black was due to a mild case of color vision confusion associated with weak rods. Jane had never been tested in school, but she knew very well that she must be colorblind. She has navy blue clothes and navy blue shoes because she has been told that this color is businesslike but not as stark as black. She has no black clothing so that she will make no mistakes. Before she had eliminated black from her wardrobe, she once arrived at work with one black and one blue shoe and a black skirt and a navy jacket. Some thought she was trying to express an original style. She noticed the problem when she bent down to pick up a dropped pencil and saw that one shoe had a bow and the other did not. Now, she also owns only solid-colored blouses, or blouses that appear to be white with some singular delicate stripe of another color. The only jewelry she wears is pearls. This, in fact, has given her a unique personal look and she is satisfied.

YELLOW COLOR VISION CONFUSION

People are taught that yellow is one of the three primary colors (the colors in Munsell's wheel as discussed on page 95). For yellow to be mistaken for white, grey, or black when it is so basic a color may be hard to accept. But late in the last century, the German physiologist Ewald Hering noted that loss of yellow color vision can happen. He also noted that yellow color vision confusion is related to blue vision disturbance.

Hering found that even non-colorblind people can have problems with yellow and blue-related color confusion. Indeed, Hering discovered that, at times, yellow and blue together will cause anyone, colorblind or not, to see white, not the expected green. This can be proven by a simple experiment that you can conduct yourself. Make a disc by cutting a circle of cardboard and punching a hole in the center. Color half of the disc blue and the other half yellow—construction paper or paint will do. Next, place this disc on top of a pen or pencil, and twirl it. As you twirl the disc, you will see what seems to be white. This "change" or "disappearance of color" can be seen by persons who have full color vision and colorblind people as well.

Hering also stated that seeing colors requires not only registering color, but also registering relative brightness. It is not surprising, therefore, that some who have trouble seeing colors are very attuned to brightness and darkness. This is one way for colorblind people to substitute visual cues.

Some Daily Problems and Adjustments

Loss of yellow vision can cause a person to see butter as lard, urine as water, some types of green as white, and sunshine as grey. It is of value, however, to sharpshooters to delete yellow vision. They actually wear yellow tinted glasses to cancel yellow in their sight so they will get a sharper image. In fact, I know a red/green colorblind sharpshooter who chose a yellow tint for his daily-wear glasses.

BLUE-YELLOW COLOR VISION CONFUSION

Inherited yellow-blue CVC is much more rare than red-green confusion, but it does happen. For people who have blue-yellow confusion, pure blue wavelengths seem to "shift" until they are confused with green. People with this type of CVC see green as blue and blue as green. They may confuse blue and green, blue and violet, dark blue and dark red, light pastel colors. In certain cases, light blue and yellow are both mistaken for white or sand color. In other cases, either blue or yellow may appear as somewhere between white and grey. Some people have more problems with the yellow end of the spectrum than with the blue. While the inability to see blue will be noted, the inability to see yellow properly is often disregarded as insignificant.

Some Daily Problems and Adjustments

As with other forms of CVC, there are some occupations that just are not suited to those with blue-yellow CVC. Becoming an electrical engineer or a boat or plane captain are generally bad ideas. These jobs require the ability to distinguish lights and wires of all colors. Any job that involves mixing chemicals and comparing them to color charts is also one to avoid. But do not be discouraged, there are jobs out there that do not involve any of these skills. Working with numbers may be an option, in accounting or bookkeeping for instance. Your areas of expertise can most likely be used toward a job that does not require color differentiation, but this is an area that most explore on their own, usually finding out by accident what jobs are not suited to them through trial and error.

There are a number of jewelers who say that blue-yellow CVC is really a boon to them because they are less distracted by the dazzle of reflected or refracted colors and can focus on minute flaws in jewelry that appear as specks or thin lines. For this reason, they can tell the quality of gold (in fact, there is "white" gold and "black" gold) far more quickly than others can. They can also determine the sparkle or flaw of a diamond very easily, though they may not be able to evaluate its color very well.

ACHROMATOPSIA

The most rare type of color vision confusion is a blindness to all colors—actual colorblindness. We do not know why achromatopsia occurs, but it afflicts one out of 33,000 people. It is associated with some problem area in the central nervous system, not the retina. Those who have achromatopsia see life in what we would call monochrome, or greys, although if you ask them, they may tell you that they see rich variations of tonalities. In fact, they often pick up visual details others would miss or dismiss.

In this condition, the photoreceptors involved in night vision remain intact, but those for day vision are almost completely absent. People who have achromatopsia, therefore, have dark-adapted vision. The rods, dealing not with colors but with tones of dark and light, become the main source of vision for these people. The number of cones in these peoples' eyes may vary, but they are either not functioning or else are so few in number so that they can hardly be effective. Why it happens is still not known, but for some it seems that the body is inhibited from generating cone cells.

A major problem with achromatopsia is that it is often misdiagnosed because the retinas of affected people look perfectly normal in an ordinary eye exam. Affected people don't seem to have any visual impairment, yet when they're asked to read an eye chart, they can do so only with much effort. Some have been accused of trying to attract attention or of being uncooperative, especially since they avoid certain activities.

Children who have this problem love to stay up at night. During the day, they are clingy and appear to be shy and fearful. In reality, without protective lenses to shield their eyes from the light, they need to be led by the hand through outdoor activities in daylight hours.

An eye chart has now been devised to test for achromatopsia, and many cases are being studied by Dr. Gunilla Haegerstrom-Portnoy, a practicing optometrist and a researcher at the School of Optometry of the University of California at Berkeley. She pinpointed why people test for achromatopsia, and her findings were announced in 1992. To pinpoint the problem and determine just how little color vision is even possible for some people, a test called an electroretinogram (ERG) has been developed to detect the absence of cone signals. In this way, even young children can be diagnosed and outfitted with the proper set of protective glasses. Again, it is helpful to be aware and to test for the disorder.

Some Daily Problems and Adjustments

One woman who has achromatopsia is a ranger at Yosemite National Park. Because of her excellent night vision and ability to spot "night critters," she leads nighttime hikes. Another person with achromatopsia worked for a while in a hospital darkroom. Neither of these people was willing to accept that they see in only black and white. Both say that they see colors in their own way, but it is not clear what they mean. Few people who have this condition offer to open up and tell their story. They have felt so intimidated for so long that they would rather not hear another negative word.

It is really hard for anyone who has full color vision to imagine living with limited color vision or constant confusion of colors. It is difficult to explain what the "colors" of the colorblindness are. Dr. Mary Collins wrote one of the few books with the colorblind person in mind. Dr. Collins was a professor of psychology and physiology at the University of Edinburgh, Scotland. In her book, *Colourblindness*, which appeared in 1925, she concluded that those who are colorblind do not guess colors. She said that these people have a definite system of color sensation that they rely on. Each develops his or her own personal system. She found they will often speak of "reddish-green," a color that people with full color vision can hardly imagine. A modification in light is often considered by a colorblind person not as a change in the tone of a color, but as a separate color altogether. I have found this to be true among people who have inherited color vision confusion as well. Could we explain to them what it is they are missing? I doubt it. Can we really feel how they manage and how they determine what is what? I doubt that, too. The most puzzling question is why this confusing situation exists. Why did nature choose to have colorblindness happen?

IN CONCLUSION

People who have full color vision are called trichromats. People who have problems seeing colors are dichromats. Some have trouble with greens or reds, others with blues or yellows. Far fewer see only in black and white, or variations of grays. These people are monochromats. There is a rare condition the causes people to be achromats—they prefer the dark. But everyone needs some degree of light in order to see. The importance of light to vision in general, and to color vision in particular, has long been overlooked as we shall see in the next chapter.

4

The Importance of Light

Light affects us all. Without light our eyes cannot see colors, whether we have the capacity for seeing the full spectrum of colors or whether we have color vision confusion. Even those who have full color vision need the proper lighting to see the chroma (intensity) and value (relative darkness or lightness) of a color. Those who have color vision confusion often rely even more heavily on the proper lighting because under some conditions they can differentiate colors, and under other conditions they confuse the colors. Spatial discrimination also depends on light. In order to figure out distance, depth, and the other factors that permit us to see in three dimensions, we need at least a little bit of light.

Consider how your eyes function while driving in a car at night. We rely on lights to give us clues about what is out there, how far away it is, and if other objects are around it. Light allows us to get a sense of location even if we do not see the whole panorama.

Light sensitivity, you will recall, is the function of the rods. But what are the lighting conditions that allow for optimum rod function? What lighting conditions are best? This has been argued for a long time. The best answer that can be given is, it all depends.

Many of you may remember that as children, you were chastised by your mothers to turn on more light in order to see properly—whether you were watching television or reading a comic book. You may have been warned that poor lighting would make you go blind. Your mothers were wrong about going blind, but they were right about the need for good lighting. However, your mothers had little knowledge of what good lighting was, and often refused to accept that lighting that may be good for one purpose may be inadequate or overkill for another.

Take, for instance, bathroom lighting fixtures. Many people use the type they imagine is used by movie or theater stars. Often people do not understand that this design—lights in a row at each side of the mirror and above the mirror—has a particular use for those who need to see how they will look with a spotlight focused on them. Actors and actresses use this style of lighting not because they are stars, but because they must pay close attention to various aspects of their facial makeup. Faces have hills and valleys, areas that cast shadows, and creases. When a spotlight, or perhaps a number of spotlights from various directions and in various colors, is focused on a performer's face, the actor might wish to subdue, highlight, or boldly emphasize the shadows and creases. Lighting is a very important way of projecting the personality of the character to the audience.

But similar lights for the activity of brushing your teeth in the morning can be considered overuse of light. This is true for those who can see the full spectrum as well as for those who are colorblind. The effect of high brightness, especially when it is reflected off a mirror directly into the eye, can be similar to that of snow blindness (erythropsia), in which you see blotches float in front of your eyes.

Few people recognize that lighting should be a major aspect in planning the interior of a building, whether a private home in the country or an office building in a busy metropolis. Unfortunately, lighting consultants, who are trained to make the environment attractive as well as functional, are rarely called in when buildings are designed, either for residential purposes or for work and study areas like schools and businesses. Much time and money is spent on selecting fixtures, but little on the use of the lighting or the needs of the people. This lack of attention is not just the fault of architects, contractors, or electricians. The client is often equally unconcerned and often ignorant of the significance of light in daily living and productivity. When it comes to the workplace, where the architects have often been told to cut corners and to streamline budgets, planning for good lighting suffers. Most developers do not care, and most of those who rent the space do not consider whether the area's design and lighting are suited for the work that will take place there. The net result for those who will use the building is uncomfortable lighting levels, and light sources that can cause headaches, nausea, poor productivity, and confusion of colors.

There is much to be considered when choosing lighting for a room. For instance, what kind of activity is intended for the area and who will use it? Is it going to be a recreational room for children or the elderly? Is it going to be a conference room in which low-key gatherings and contract deals will be consummated, or a conference room that will rely heavily on slides, video tapes, and other visual displays?

Other aspects of room lighting also affect those with CVC differently. If you've ever looked at the bright light of the window for about five minutes and then looked away, you may have noticed that you see the rectangular design of the window floating before your eyes. Similarly, if you have full color vision and were to concentrate on a red light, you would see a green blob floating before your eyes when you looked away. If you concentrated on a green light, you would see red after turning your eyes away. Those who have red-green CVC can note the "negative" of the rectangular window, but they cannot see afterimages in color—either the red or the green floating negative.

Have you ever seen pink and green iridescent highlights on a soap bubble although nothing green or pink was nearby to reflect in the bubble? These colors that have no "real" basis seem to be out of the range of people who have red-green CVC.

Even people who have full color vision may be tricked. Consider, for instance, a scene composed of snow and sky. If you put a mirror on the snow and allow the sky to reflect into it, you would find that the sky is brighter than the snow.

But for some people, light may often spell the difference between seeing a color and not seeing it. Dr. Leo Hurwich, who has done a significant amount of research on the subject of light, tells of an employee at Eastman Kodak many years ago, who was always teased about his confused color vision. His frustration drove him to Hurwich's lab where he was tested by Dr. Hurwich and a Professor Jameson. It turned out that he could see colors fine as long as the light was adjusted to a different intensity than others needed. Imagine trying to tune into a radio station when your dial is broken. To receive the transmission, you must adjust it to a slightly different position in order to receive the frequency clearly. This man needed to have the light adjusted in order to receive the right color information. He was euphoric when his problem and the light adjustments were explained to him. In fact, the other employees were dumfounded when they discovered that under the adjusted light, this man could match colors better than they could.

Recently, I found a similar case. This man is the color reproduction matcher I prefer to deal with at the local Kinko's in Greenville, North Carolina. Other employees there have often joked about his color vision, and are stunned when I insist that he handle my orders. They were stunned when he proved that he can match colors better than they can when I dared them to compete. He says he has his own private compensating system.

Sometimes people do not admit to the significance of inappropriate lighting, like the disturbance bright light can cause, or the dissatisfaction low light can generate. Consider how easily we accept the dangers of momentary blindness from the lights of oncoming cars. Such blindness as you sit behind the wheel of a vehicle moving forward toward potential disaster can be scary enough to literally cause a heart attack. If more people spoke up, the automobile industry would make changes. Lights that do not cause such blindness are available and not expensive. In fact, in the 1930s, Edwin Land designed polarized sheets of plastic that were colorless and transparent. This plastic was not meant for sunglasses, but for use in headlights of cars. The American automobile industry did not buy the sheets then, and has not bought them yet.

As frightening as it may sound, most red colorblind people cannot see a danger signal presented as a red light. Thankfully, amber lights have now been introduced for the back lights and for turn lights. At night, amber lights can be seen by all, those who have full color vision and those who are colorblind. Until recently, amber lights were not as prevalent, and one could find them only mainly on foreign cars. This was due to the fact that, in the 1960s, auto accidents on the German roadways were very common. The passenger side of the front seats had become known by then as the "death seat." The roadways were free of speed limits; speeding and "free-wheeling" behavior was seen as youthful zeal and an expression of freedom from the oppressive Nazi era. In addition, medicine was nationalized, which meant that if you did get hurt, your medical needs would be taken care of by the government of Germany. Both the car insurance industry and the nationalized medical services became fed up and decided to find a solution to whiplash injuries and front-end damages that resulted. Serious efforts were made to find out how to reduce tail-end collisions. The amber taillights did the trick.

Amber lights made such a difference that it was decided to test many young adults for colorblindness. It turned out that a far larger number had red vision confusion than the examiners expected. Most of these drivers, the majority of whom were in their early 30s and 40s, had never been tested for color vision.

From that time on, all cars made in Germany were required to have amber lights in back. This was also expected of the Ford products that were assembled in Germany. I am told that this change made a significant difference in the cost of carrying the national medical program. Costs of dealing with hospital care, mortuary care, rehabilitation, and home care dropped significantly simply because there were fewer accidents, and those that did occur were not as serious.

In the past twenty years, all Japanese-made cars have also had amber taillights. Few American-made cars did. The sale of American cars dropped dramatically for various reasons in the 1980s, and many felt that American cars were less safe. One of the reasons may have been that American cars provided fewer clues for seeing cars in the darkness of night, especially on poorly lit roads like those in rural areas.

You may have noticed that you rarely hear of whiplash injuries these days, not because they do not occur at all, but because their occurrence is much more seldom. Trucks are equipped with amber lights on all sides. (You will also find this color on road work warning signals, such as cones, and on construction safety gear, such as helmets.) The color that some call amber and others call orange appears as red or green or some other definite, noticeable color to most who have red/green CVC.

Of course, outdoors, light cannot be controlled. You can do little about day turning to night, or the shadow of a building falling on an area. What about sunglasses? Sunglasses do not always do the job we think they do. In 1991, researchers tried to find out whether people would have fewer accidents, especially when the glare of the sun is greatest, if they wore sunglasses. The answer was a surprising "No." The researchers found that sunglasses do not prevent accidents. Why? For one thing, people who wear sunglasses often choose them for cosmetic reasons. Most people who choose glasses in this category find that the glasses do very little to cut down glare. Such sunglasses are actually unsuitable—possibly even dangerous—for driving. What's more, when sunglasses are worn, the pupils of driver's eyes dilate as they would at night to adjust to the shade the glasses give. The eyes then tire more easily, which could be dangerous to the driver. This phenomenon is not mentioned in advertisements or in any public forum.

Light also plays a strong role in depth perception. If you look at a mile-long row of electrical poles along a road, you find that they appear to get smaller in the distance and that they look white or are a different color than the poles closest to you. The color is based on the amount of dark coloration surrounding the poles. None of the poles may be in shadow and all may be equally lit, but your eyes will register them differently.

People with red-green CVC cannot see certain "tricks" of light at all. The colored lights involved in such atmospheric happenings as rainbows and halos around the moon (like the previously mentioned soap bubbles) are completely lost on those who are colorblind. These colors are created by the refraction of lights rather than by pigment—the actual color of the "skin" of the object.

In other cases, people need very little light. This is true for people who have achromatopsia—complete colorblindness in which only gray in varying degrees of luminosity is seen (see page 36). It is also true for those who have blue-cone monochromy. The eyes of the people in both groups are dark-adapted or sensitive to light. The affected people are happier with the light of dawn or dusk, or even night. Daylight hurts their eyes. Their vision works best primarily in low light. In bright light, they must look through tinted lenses. Admittedly, there are not many such people but, as you will find in Chapter 5, acquired rod damage can cause such a condition.

One of the earliest such cases was reported in 1684, about the time the Pilgrims landed on Plymouth Rock. *The Philosophical Transactions of the Royal Society of London* reported the case of a woman of "three and twenty years who could see no colors." She could, however, read in the dark for almost a quarter of an hour (probably by the light of the moon).

A Case of Acquired Light Sensitivity

In a more recent case, an industrial construction field engineer became sensitive to light after being struck on her eye during a marital argument. An optometrist suggested that the lenses this woman had previously worn to correct nearsightedness be tinted brown to help her adjust to bright light. The brown tinting caused migraine headaches for which the medication Ergomar was prescribed. This caused nausea and an increased aversion to light. The tint was then darkened without benefit.

Following her divorce, the woman moved to another town where she found an optometrist who offered a solution. First, he tried grey lenses, which, she said, caused "things to just not look right." After trying a blue tint that caused mild nausea, purple lenses were tried. But purple did not eliminate all of the glare. Now, she wears lenses that are tinted 20 percent brown and 20 percent purple and are quite dark. She is, however, still able to work. She has to work from memory to adjust to the dark world she now lives in through her new lenses. Although people who wear sunglasses do the same thing, this woman has to do so indoors, too. In addition, she has tinted safety glasses to use when welding and doing other work. These glasses had to be specially approved by the Occupational Safety and Health Administration (OSHA) since its maximum approved level of tinting is only 15 percent.

This woman used to see colors and light in full. Now, because of her injury, she must wear tinted glasses during the day, and she can see colors only at dusk and twilight. At other times, she is forced to see colors in a distorted way if she is to see at all.

Current Lighting Research

Despite the importance of light to human life, research on lighting has only recently become a serious study. Since 1990, astronauts have been receiving "light treatment" to help their biological rhythms adjust to their being awake during late-night hours. Accurately timed exposure to bright light can disrupt the body's circadian rhythms, which regulate such biological processes as body temperature fluctuation, heart rate, and the sleep-wake cycle. Scientists now know that a cluster of 10,000 neurons (the suprachiasmatic nucleus or SCN) located on the hypothalamus, reacts to light and darkness by sending messages to other parts of the brain and body.

This light treatment—known as phototherapy—is also being used to treat age-related sleep problems. According to the National Institute on Aging, more than half of those over sixty-five experience some sleeping difficulty such as waking too early. Scientists surmise that the circadian pacemaker speeds up as people age. By the age of sixty-five, a person will sleep from 10 p.m. to 6 a.m. instead of sleeping from 11 p.m. to 7 a.m. and may have trouble staying awake until 10 p.m. by the age of seventy. When older people are exposed to bright light during the early evening hours, the sleep-wake cycle seems to be delayed.

Sometimes, light is used to treat emotional problems. People who suffer from seasonal affective disorder (SAD), experience abnormal sleep patterns, fatigue, withdrawal, and depression usually when the days grow shorter in the fall and winter. When sufferers are exposed to fluorescent lights at 2,500 lux (ordinarily, room light is 500 lux or less) for two hours each day, depression lifts even among severely depressed patients.

Now that light is becoming a topic of serious study, people are studying the use of lighting in such fields as crime prevention, job satisfaction, and marketing. For instance, vegetables are being displayed in supermarkets with focused lighting so they will look fresher. The use of light to enhance appearance of products at trade fairs has also been investigated. Insurance companies are conducting research into the use of lighting to decrease accidents. Light, you see, has been found to be crucial for the "bottom line" so to speak—it has financial implications. Hopefully, researchers will investigate not only how to get the best lighting for the money but how light affects color perception. Computer use is one of the most fertile areas for study.

Computers and Light

Consider, if you will, that most buildings were not built with consideration of the computer users who would be inside. Even if sufficient electric wires and outlets were installed to accommodate computers, appropriate illumination for those who work with computer terminals was often ignored.

In recent years, there has been increasing interest in how the light from computers affects viewers. People have to deal with computer monitors at work as well as in school and at home, even for playing games. No wonder those interested in productivity are concerned about the effects of sitting in one location, watching one small area on which letters move and lights are flashed.

These people know that the light in which people work, and the glare projected from computer screens can affect sight. Architects were among the first to notice that eye fatigue can develop easily when the environmental light is not compatible with the light on computer screens. Architects, who were early users of computer graphics as models for developing architectural and horticultural plans, labeled the problem "stare glare." Stare glare leads to a gradual decline in performance. The effect is similar to that of low lighting, which causes a decline in performance because with little light, little is recorded by the eye.

The computer monitor is very different than a page of paper. The use of color was once limited and carefully considered because reproduction of colors was so expensive. This is no longer the case. Now we have an overload of color, presented in a indiscriminate manner that abuses the senses. Furthermore, a page of paper is white, and written material contrasts with it, appearing in a darker hue, be it black or some color. On a monochrome computer monitor, the background is often a dark color or black, and the material on it appears in white. Black on white is clearer to the eye than is white on color. What's more, if the screen is black, the blackness commands our attention first, then the letters or designs on it.

This harks back to what Goethe was studying (see Chapter 7). He was dealing with light as "read" against the dark, and to what extent that light can be manipulated for stage effects. But working at a computer is not like being in an audience at a stage performance. In the interactive world of computers, you often have to follow colored signals or cues to make the computer move on to a subsequent step.

Some of the earliest research on how light from computer screens effects vision was conducted at the Eye Research Laboratory of the University of Chicago. Researchers also considered the problems that can occur when colors are used on a computer screen without regard to viewer reaction to those colors. The investigators noted how confusing the colors on a computer screen can be to a colorblind person. But no effort was made to determine how many producers of computer graphics have CVC. Nor did anyone consider how confusing graphics produced by such people might be to others.

Once the computer field was a haven for the colorblind. Computer people had to understand how to program and had to deal with logic more than with visual communication. For this reason, many who entered the field at first were not visual communicators but physicists and mathematicians. Many who program graphics still have no background in cognitive psychology (the study of such mental tasks as perception, reasoning, and judgment and the processes that permit their performance). They may know little about the significance of design placement, variations of texture and color use.

An organization known as SIGGRAPH was founded in Chicago by the developer of C-GRAPH software program for computer-generated color graphics use, Thomas Di Fanti. SIGGRAPH has existed for more than twenty years and is considered the premier place to display new developments of computer-generated color graphics. Dr. Di Fanti is also the founder of the University of Illinois Electronic Visualization Lab in Chicago. He has been a leader in the study of misuse of colors, willful confusion of colors, and colors chosen poorly for coding information. He is also an advocate of using textural effects in conjunction with colors. He has long called for the restraint of "aesthetics." By this he means visual sensibility, or sensitivity to the fact that misuse of color and design can be insulting, abusive, and downright counterproductive in industrial and educational settings where computer use is strong.

This is especially important in respect to the prevalent use of computer-generated maps. Color use on computerized maps can lead to misreading, even for those who are sure they can differentiate between blue and green. For the colorblind, the use of red for major highways constitutes a loss of information because if they see it, they see it as black, as black as any other road or county line.

Another computer problem many people have to deal with at work is that colors on computer monitors may not be the colors that are output by the printer. This is confusing for those who see colors, and even more so for those who have doubts about the colors they see in the first place. Problems are compounded by the fact that much display information on computer monitors is still poorly designed, although there have been great strides since Apple, the first personal computer, was introduced to homes and industry in 1977.

And now motion is being used in abundance. "Zip-zap" visuals are everywhere. The colored moving lights can take fantastic turns and form shapes without limit to the level of virtual reality. Such graphics can be beneficial, but can also be harmful if misused. And this new technology is sweeping the world, even entering hospital operating rooms where split-second decisions are based on computer-generated images. Just consider, then, how necessary it is to understand the effects of the colors used, as well as their clarity, given the lighting conditions of the operating table and the visual capacities of the viewer.

And let's not forget that even computers can be colorblind. The

United States Postal Service has had its share of such problems when using computers to sort mail. The difficulties are most obvious at Christmastime when green ink is used on white or yellow envelopes, or black ink is used on red envelopes that must be sorted by machine. The colors used on cards or gifts to enhance the holiday spirit cause computers to "go down" and give up.

Eventually, someone will improve the program that gives instruction to the postal computers. People, you know, can program computers but humans are not programmed. They simply have to contend with their existing capacity for color vision.

IN CONCLUSION

As you can see, lighting conditions have a great impact on how well people can see colors, especially those with CVC. With a little attention given to fixtures, and a little thought given to usage, correct lighting can help us all.

5

Causes of Color Vision Confusion

You may now be thinking that although color vision confusion is a problem, you needn't worry. You are not colorblind. Consider, however, that there are several ways a person can become colorblind. CVC can be acquired as well as inherited. Even though the vast majority of known cases of color vision confusion are inherited, the number of cases of acquired CVC is increasing drastically for reasons you will soon understand.

While most people who inherit CVC confuse red and green, those who acquire CVC most often—but not always—confuse the blue-yellow range of colors. A major reason for the blue color vision problem in acquired cases is that the cones that react to short wavelengths are more sensitive to injury and chemical changes in the body than the cones that aid us in seeing red.

Under normal conditions, blue is the easiest color to see because this color's wavelength has the shortest route to the eye. Thus, for those who have inherited color vision confusion, the additional loss of the one "assured" color is traumatic indeed.

Because most cases of CVC are inherited, let's start with a very brief explanation of how traits in general are inherited.

A GENETICS PRIMER

The information in each of our cells came to us when our mother's and father's sex cells (the sperm and the ovum) joined to develop the first cell from which our bodies formed. We inherit all physical characteristics from our parents. Each bit of information—whether it's about the makeup of an earlobe or the size of a foot—is transferred from the parent to the child through a gene. For each trait, there are two genes; these paired genes are called alleles. These genes can be compared to beads. Chromosomes are strings of these beads. The beaded strings appear in the form of an X or Y when viewed under a microscope. Females normally have XX chromosomes in their cells and males have XY.

Each of the sex cells contains half the necessary genetic information. In other words, each mature sex cell contains half of the pair of alleles. When a sperm cell unites with the ovum, the fertilized egg receives one allele from each parent. Genetic information determines such things as hair color, width of your nose, eye color, height, and many other details. Even the sex of the new child is determined by inherited genes. A fertilized egg must receive an X gene from the mother. The father then either contributes a Y chromosome to create a male baby (XY), or an X to create a female baby (XX).

Colorblindness is considered a sex-linked characteristic because the gene appears only on the X chromosome. If a woman inherits X genes for colorblindness from her father and normal X genes from her mother, she is only a carrier, and she can transmit it to her son because a male has both an X and a Y chromosome. The mother may not even know she is a carrier because she may not show any signs of CVC. If, however, the chromosome that she inherited from her mother has a faulty gene for color vision and she inherits a faulty X chromosome from her father, then she will be colorblind.

ACQUIRED CVC

Although it was once believed that colorblindness could occur only through heredity, it is now known that the condition can be acquired. Those with acquired CVC may experience any of the kinds of color confusion described in Chapter 3. However, certain color vision disturbances are experienced only by those with acquired CVC. Some cases are temporary, some are permanent. Listed here are cases of temporary CVC, which is generally called *chromatopsia*.

• *Chloropsia*—a condition in which all objects appear yellow. This condition often is a result of an overdose or high dose of digitalis (see page 65). The condition should go away once use of the drug is discontinued.

• *Cyanopsia*—a condition in which all objects appear to be blue. This condition may temporarily follow cataract surgery (see page 54).

• *Erythropsia*—a condition in which all objects appear to be tinged in red. People have reported experiencing this condition as a result of "snow blindness," in which the sun's rays are reflected and amplified by the snow. Sunglasses that protect against ultra violet light (and few really do so) can protect against erythropsia.

• *Xanthopsia*—a condition in which all objects appear yellow. This condition occurs with overdoses of picric (used as an application for burns) and some hypertension drugs. This condition will also go away once use of the drug is discontinued.

FACTORS THAT LEAD TO ACQUIRED COLORBLINDNESS

So far we have discussed at great length how a person can inherit color vision confusion. As awareness of CVC increases, awareness of cases of acquired CVC has also increased. Listed here are factors that can lead to acquired colorblindness.

1. Chronic illnesses
2. Trauma that damages the head or eye
3. Glare of sun, snow, or sea
4. Side effects of medications, alcoholism, and drug abuse
5. Toxic fumes and other industrial irritants
6. The natural process of aging

Although there may be other reasons, in this book we will examine only these common occurrences.

Illnesses

There are a number of illnesses that are known to cause color vision confusion. Some of those you are sure to recognize are:

Alzheimer's disease. It has been hard to test Alzheimer's patients for the incidence of color loss due to visual or neural problems, because their responses are not reliable. Colors, which are learned and are also triggers of memory, become confused. Loss of color vision or color memory is particularly disturbing for these patients because they are often confused enough without the additional change in their visual world.

Cataracts. Although this condition may cause people to see the world through a red film, this is not technically a case of chromatopsia. In reality, those with cataracts are seeing the world through their own blood vessels. Once the cataract is removed, this film disappears. Cyanopsia (blue CVC) may, however, temporarily occur following removal of the cataract. In one case, a patient reported blue-yellow vision disturbance three months after a cataract operation. However, the condition was the result of an infection associated with the use of contact lenses.

People who have lens implants following cataract surgery often speak glowingly of the new color sight that they experience. An ophthalmologist who had the implant in one eye spoke of seeing the flame in a gas jet as a brilliant blue with his "new eye." With his other eye, the flame appeared a grey-green-blue. In addition, his "new eye" saw the saturation of red at sunset more vividly. Porcelain appeared a brilliant violet-white with that eye, while it looked simply white with the other. Greens seemed to be bluer, and blues seemed to lean more toward purple.

Childhood diseases. Whooping cough and measles (both of which can be avoided through immunization) are two of the childhood diseases that can cause temporary color vision confusion. In whooping cough, extreme spastic coughing may cause blood vessels in the eyes or brain to burst. Fortunately, the blood vessels can regenerate after the person has recovered from the disease, and color vision can return.

Measles can make the rods in the retina so sensitive that light is uncomfortable and color differentiation is difficult. A person with measles should remain in a darkened room. This sensitivity will subside with the symptoms of the disease.

Not too long ago, these diseases were nearly eradicated, but rates of occurrence are increasing because people are not using available vaccines.

Diabetes. When a person has had diabetes (a disease involving problems digesting, metabolizing, and absorbing glucose) for more than ten years, color vision loss sometimes occurs.

Diabetes-related CVC was determined after extensive testing was conducted in Finland in 1988. These tests revealed that diabetic children will often not exhibit any CVC. This testing was conducted in Finland because there is an unusually high incidence of diabetes among young children there. (Diabetes affects the lives of 28.6 children per 100,000 annually in Finland; in the United States, 14.7 children per 100,000 annually are affected; and in Japan, only .8 per 100,000 annually are affected). Other research has confirmed that fewer diabetic children than adults are affected by blue-color vision disability.

But, it is estimated that 30 to 70 percent of the adult diabetic population has some color vision disturbance. Usually, color vision defects are associated with the development of *retinopathy*, which causes cone damage. Retinopathy is a condition in which the retina is damaged due to ocular or systemic vascular disorders. Veins in the eye become inflamed and twisted and retinal hemorrhages may occur. Retinopathy is particularly severe in those suffering from insulin-dependent diabetes mellitus (IDDM) and is frequent with chronic non-insulin-dependent diabetes mellitus (NIDDM). This is particularly disturbing since many diabetic patients rely on their color vision for interpreting color-based urine or blood glucose tests administered at home. The American Diabetes Association suggests that diabetics could avoid color vision loss by altering their lifestyles to cope with the disease and by taking such preventive measures as monitoring medication and nutrition carefully.

Glaucoma. Another eye condition that can cause color vision distortion, glaucoma may decrease a person's sensitivity to blue-green-yellow colors and tends to cause seeing "halos" around lights.

Leukemia, Addison's disease, and pernicious anemia. These conditions also can lead to CVC. Older individuals who suffer from these conditions seem less able to discriminate among purple, blue, and green.

Liver diseases. Among the liver conditions that cause CVC is cirrhosis of the liver. In this case, the CVC due to cirrhosis can often be reversed if the person reduces the consumption of alcoholic beverages, the major cause of this disease. Cirrhosis of the liver, like a number of liver diseases, interferes with absorption of vitamin A, a fat-soluble vitamin that is found in many foods including green leafy vegetables, tomatoes, and carrots. Without vitamin A, the retina cannot function properly and the rods and cones cannot be repaired and maintained.

The photosensitive pigment of the rods and the cones is formed from vitamin A in combination with the protein opsin. If the rods and cones do not receive these nutrients on a regular basis, preferably by way of the foods that we eat, they do not function properly.

That liver diseases can cause color vision confusion was first reported by Guy Verriest in 1964. It is interesting to note that alcoholism has been determined to have a genetic basis, and that the gene associated with the addictive tendency is located near the gene for color vision on the long arm of the X chromosome. We may yet discover a connection between the two conditions. Ironically, one of the medications given for alcoholism is disulfiram, which can cause red-green confusion (see page 65).

Chronic alcoholism. Since 1965, tests have shown that at least 50 percent of chronic alcoholics suffer from color vision loss or confusion. Most recently, some interesting new observations of the effects of alcohol on color vision were made in a test conducted by the Department of Psychiatry of the University Hospital of Vienna, Austria.

The University Hospital test showed that full color vision is restored when alcohol consumption is stopped. However, it also showed that there are some factors in just how well and how quickly someone will regain color vision if drinking is stopped. For one, it depends whether the consumption of alcohol was done in conjunction with other chemical substances. And, the return of color vision depends on just how much liver damage had been caused by chronic drinking.

In most cases, full color vision returned after eleven days of abstaining from drinking any alcoholic beverage. Some showed significant changes in vision after only one week. Some needed three weeks for full color vision to return.

Macular degeneration. Those affected by macular degeneration may experience color confusion along with deterioration in overall vision. Macular degeneration is an eye problem in which there is degeneration of a spot on the retina near the optic nerve, the macula lutea. It

---

WHAT'S YOUR FAVORITE COLOR?

Some psychological conditions are also linked to color vision distur-
bances. These disturbances are not connected with any problems
involving the rods and cones in the eye, but seem to be linked with the
chemical imbalances that cause the conditions.

Schizophrenics tend to adore white and will sometimes act as though
no other color exists. One test revealed that only 29 percent of the peo-
ple who are considered mentally stable prefer white, but 76.6 percent of
the schizophrenics tested preferred white.

Some people who suffer from clinical depression, which has been
shown to have a physiological basis, have reported that they not only
feel blue, but they see things as if through a blue haze.

Perhaps these observances regarding color and mental stability can
help clinicians gain some insight into how different chemical imbalances
affect color perception. Therapy using color may even be used in the
future to "balance" certain conditions. If nothing else, awareness of how
psychological conditions affect color vision can be an aid in diagnosis.

---

most often happens in association with general aging, but it may be
inherited or caused by tuberculosis.

Multiple sclerosis (MS) and Parkinson's disease. In Parkinson's disease, nerve and brain cells die, but in MS the sheath that protects
nerve cells wears away and causes "electrical shorting" of the "inner
telephone" lines of the body. With both Parkinson's and MS, there is
a breakdown in communication between nerve cells. Victims of MS
experience all sorts of visual disturbances and some eventually
become totally blind. Blurred vision and loss of color vision are clues
in the diagnosis of MS.

Retinitis pigmentosa. Often referred to as RP, this condition causes
degeneration of the retina, leading to loss of color vision and eventually to blindness. The first sign of this inherited disease is the onset of
night blindness or an inability to see in dimly lit places. The gene for
the condition is carried by one out of eighty people and seems to
occur most often among those of Irish descent.

A group of researchers led by Peter Humphries of Trinity College of Dublin, and a group working at Harvard Medical School, have been studying the disorder. They have discovered a link between the ability to see purple and the occurrence of retinitis pigmentosa. It appears that a defect in one of the color vision genes that helps to distinguish purple appears in about 30 percent of the cases of retinitis pigmentosa. The cause for many of the other cases of eye diseases has also recently been found so that research on prenatal genetic counseling can now take place.

Sickle cell anemia. In this blood ailment, found most often among African-Americans, blood cells that are normally round and donut-shaped take on a curved or C-shape. The sickle cells multiply and eventually displace the good blood cells. In the capillaries, the narrowest blood vessels, which are plentiful in the eyes, the abundance of sickle cells leads to vision problems.

The Sickle Cell Division of the National Institutes of Health, in Bethesda, Maryland, reports that patients may experience problems with colors in the blue-yellow range, but that there may be other color confusion as well. Sickle cell anemia actually destroys some of the blue vision cones, especially in the peripheral range. A major problem in diagnosing this development is that the physical changes in the eye that cause the color vision confusion cannot easily be detected by a family physician, who may dismiss the complaint.

Loss or impairment of color vision may be a side effect of other illness as well. Remember, however, that some people may suffer CVC while others with the same illness may not.

Trauma

Accidents caused by physiological events, nature, or people—generally referred to as trauma—can also lead to CVC. A stroke (a blood clot or bleeding in the brain that causes a lack of oxygen) may, for instance, cause color vision loss. In some cases, this loss is temporary, while in others it may be permanent. The first reported case of stroke-related CVC was detailed in 1881. A printer reported dizziness and blindness from which he later recovered, but he suffered a loss of color vision unless the colors were seen under certain lighting conditions. When his vision first returned, the printer described light green, yellow, and blue as dirty white; pink as red; and purple as very dark. A year later, he could identify a larger number of colors, although he still could not distinguish green and could clearly identify only red and yellow.

In another case, a woman who was past eighty began to see both blue and yellow as white. Green became yellow. Far away from her family in a nursing home in the countryside, the woman was particularly bothered by her confusion about colors. She had always delighted in nature and now could not tell the seasons by the color of the lawn or the trees. She feared she was losing her mind.

One of the woman's sons came to visit during dinner hour and reported that his mother was becoming "strange." She had, for instance, used her chicken soup to clean her hands, assuming that the soup was water in a finger bowl. A doctor was called in. After examining the woman, he decided that she had had a small stroke, which had not affected her mind but had affected her color vision.

Other kinds of brain and neural damage, including concussions, can lead to spells of color vision loss. In some cases, the condition can be permanent. In one concussion case, an individual reported intermittent and temporary achromatopsia. The person felt as if he were switching to black and white television and then reverting to color while watching a single scene.

Another interesting case of CVC caused by a concussion is recounted in *An Anthropologist on Mars* by Dr. Oliver Sacks, a neurologist who has become well known for his books about unusual human conditions due to brain damage. The first case mentioned in *An Anthropologist on Mars* is of a painter who suffered a concussion from an automobile accident. After the accident, the painter thought that when he painted he used the same colors that he used before his concussion. But that was not true. In fact, he painted mainly in variations of browns and greys. This man did not sense any loss of color vision. Moreover, he would become annoyed if anyone suggested that he was not painting in the full range of colors.

As Dr. Sacks recalls, immediately after the painter's accident and for a year or more thereafter, the painter insisted that he "knew" colors. He knew what was beautiful, what was appropriate, but that was all in his mind. As time went by, the painter had to admit that he was less and less sure of the colors he was seeing. His behavior began to resemble that of someone who was born colorblind, even though he had lived in a world of color for his first sixty-one years.

What happened next was quite interesting. This painter became dazzled by the sight of very bright lights. He veered more and more toward a night-life. He found it more comfortable to walk in the street at dusk or at night. By the time this man was sixty-five, four years after the accident, he reported, "My vision is such that everything on television looks black and white to me. . . . I can see a worm wriggling a block away. The sharpness of focus is incredible." How it is that one kind of vision was exchanged for another is still a mystery.

In another accident, a colorblind marine who landed on an electrical wire after he had parachuted from a plane reported that "everything turned bright, flaming yellow. Thunderbolts seemed to ricochet through me." His color vision had returned.

Nature can also cause traumatic injuries that disturb color vision. A man who had been stung in the eye saw one set of colors with that eye and other colors when looking through the uninjured eye.

Glare

The sun's harsh reflection off sand, sea, or snow can cause temporary or permanent CVC, depending on the duration and intesity of the reflection. This is not an uncommon way for people in professions that keep them outdoors for long periods of time to acquire CVC.

Some military personnel who served in the Desert Storm campaign in 1991 appear to have an acquired color vision problem that has yet to be diagnosed. The problem may be the result of their looking at burning Iraqi oil wells and holding tanks for long periods of time. The fires set by soldiers from Kuwait lasted for weeks on end and caused a film of soot to fill the air. In addition, troops were not warned of potential eye damage from prolonged exposure to the sun's glare on the desert sands. Sunglasses were optional. Yet we have known about the loss of color vision associated with the desert sun for more than fifty years.

Shortly before World War II, British medical personnel in the area then known as Palestine noticed that Beduin men seemed to have defective color vision. The discovery was made because, in an attempt to surmount the language barrier, color-coded signs were used to denote borders, areas in which camels were allowed to be left, areas where water was available, and the location of various offices. The colors seemed to be a simple solution to the communication problem until it was shown that most of the Beduins who roamed in the Negev—the area between the Dead Sea and the Sinai Desert—were colorblind.

At first it was assumed that the condition was the result of *trachoma*, an infectious eye disease that has plagued the Arab world for centuries. It was, however, found that the women did not have CVC. If the men had trachoma, the women would have had it, too. Another explanation had to be found.

Investigators realized that both Beduin boys and girls could see colors well. Males and females had apparently been born with the capacity for full color sight. The girls, however, had been kept at home, and when they grew into women, they wore veils. The boys, though, had been allowed to play outside. When they grew into men, they spent most of their time outdoors, scanning the desert sands and sky. The damage caused by exposure to the sun's glare became permanent.

During World War II, American troops fighting the Italian Fascist forces in the Sahara Desert region in North Africa were issued sunglasses with polarized lenses developed by Edwin Land. They were also warned about the glare of the sun on the sand. This information was somehow lost by the 1990s, and members of the generation of sun worshippers had no idea about the dangers of the desert to which they were sent.

Few troops who served in Desert Storm have spoken up about color vision confusion. Many are afraid of becoming the victims of military "down-sizing." They keep quiet because reserve activity means an extra paycheck and some fringe benefits for their families.

At least one reserve officer has, however, told me that since serving in Desert Storm, he has had a hard time seeing blue and yellow. This is rather unfortunate, especially since he has inherited red-green color vision confusion. He could always rely on his capacity to see blues before. Now he confuses blues, greens, yellows; and sometimes yellows, browns, and reds; or yellow and white.

He never gave the matter too much thought until he began to hear complaints from his troops as well. Each has had some odd experience due to loss of color vision, and each kept it to himself until it became annoying. The number of men who reported a problem seeing colors after duty surprised him. No one has yet explained to him why so many men seemed to be affected in this way. He has also wondered if the many women who were stationed in the desert were equally affected.

MEDICINE: CURE OR CAUSE?

I have personally observed one case of acquired color vision confusion at close range. My husband, Abner, began to lose color vision after being given a series of experimental medications for sudden acute hypertension. This happened in the mid 1970s when Abner was forty-two years old.

Abner had been told to lose weight and to give up smoking but found it difficult to do either. Otherwise healthy and athletic, he was a tall husky man with a physique like a football player. It did not seem dangerous for him to become a test case for new hypertension medications, and he was only too willing. You see, some thirty years earlier, his older sister had been given experimental doses of vitamin B when she was hospitalized, crippled, and nearly blind from multiple sclerosis. After receiving megadoses of the vitamin, she regained sight as well as stamina.

Because of his size, Abner was given large doses of various medications, all in conjunction with Lasix. Each was prescribed for a certain period of time—three weeks to two months in duration—unless he reacted negatively, in which case, another drug was prescribed.

From the beginning, all the medications made him dizzy and impaired the clarity of his vision. He was told that the medications might cause some disorientation in the first few days of testing, but the problem persisted and worsened.

Because Abner was so nearsighted that he had been classified 4F (not eligible for military service), I had always selected bathing suits for myself in loud colors and patterns so that I would be a visible sign-post as I waited by the pool or on the seashore while he swam. Abner loved to swim but could not tell where shore or poolside was without his glasses. He had even learned to dive with his glasses tucked next to his body in one hand so that they would be available when he played with his children in the pool. When in the ocean or doing laps in the pool, he swam without his glasses. These glasses were so much a part of him that when contact lenses became available, he chose not to try them; he felt he "heard better" with his glasses on.

Once Abner started using the test medications, whatever clear vision he had began playing tricks on him. With each succeeding medication, his vision seemed more limited, but his own awareness of color vision loss was very gradual. What bothered him most at first were the spots, stripes, and blurriness he saw. Later, he began to feel that something else was wrong with his vision, but he could not really say what. He hesitated saying anything at first because he was afraid that he was losing his mind, and he feared upsetting me.

At this time, he was seeing brilliant halos and was less and less sure of the colors of his ties and suits. He began wearing green-blue ties or ties with green stripes, although he had avoided that color before. He was even uncertain about foods. He could not distinguish one marmalade from another by color. He was repulsed by the appearance of butter. He thought his hand tools were broken because the red indicator lights no longer appeared lit when the tools were plugged in.

Had he asked his doctor about the problem? Yes, he had mentioned it, and the doctor suggested it was all in his mind, it was all part of the stress that had probably caused his hypertension in the first place.

I saw the change for myself. I knew how well he had been able to distinguish colors before. Now, he was groping to match suit and tie. He had become disoriented when taking walks at night. He would not cross a street in the evening without me by his side to tell him when the light was green. The once outgoing, distinguished-looking, and forceful trial lawyer began to lose confidence. Now, he wanted me nearby at all times, as a visual guide.

I decided to conduct a test of my own. My husband had loved to watch me paint ever since we met in college, where I was an art student and he was a student of government and law. He did not, however, like for me to use black, which he felt indicated death and sorrow. He was always eager to see me happy. Now, I was painting a series of landscapes of nearby locales using only one hue, stretching its capacities with the variations of values, using white to make the hue lighter and lighter. When Abner would come by to watch me paint, I managed to test his color vision. I would not ask him what colors were being used, but rather what he thought of the development of the painting. He knew that I usually painted with a full color palate, and that I produced impressionistic work that was filled with a sense of atmosphere, be it mist, crisp sunset, or whatever. Abner assumed I was painting with a full spectrum of colors and told me what he thought the colors were. He was way off! His selections were remembered probabilities, not what was there.

Now, I decided to speak with Abner's doctor, although I normally did not get involved. In fact, Abner had specifically asked me to accompany him on his next visit to the doctor. I asked the doctor if the medicine could cause color vision confusion. He responded that I should stop being an overprotective wife and that perhaps I was one of the major causes of my husband's hypertension.

My desire to let others know what can happen to color vision and how it can affect people's lives began that very moment.

I did not know then, nor did Abner, that the pharmaceutical industry had already been investigating digoxin toxicity after an error had been made in manufacturing the drug in 1969. In fact, Abner was part of research to re-evaluate dose levels. But neither he nor I was ever informed of that, and I only discovered the facts as I prepared the final chapters of this book. The doctor who gave him this medication had been the chief of internal medicine at French Hospital in New York City, which closed less than three years after my husband died in 1977. This doctor has never exchanged a single spoken word with me since that one day at his office.

It is not that I object to medications or to testing on humans. There are times when medication is the only course of action in order to help a patient recover from an illness or have a better quality of life. But patients and their loved ones should be given more information about potential color vision loss or confusion. Doctors must become more alert to the fact that color vision is an important source of information. They should realize that loss or confusion of color vision by a person who has had full color vision can be distracting, at best, and may be disorienting to the point that it can trigger depression or paranoia.

Today, pharmacists do give a description of side effects when a person picks up prescribed medication. This was not the case in the 1970s. Frequently, even these descriptions do not tell the whole story. You should take responsibility for your own well-being and learn about the medications that may affect your color vision.

Medications

A number of frequently used medications may cause color vision confusion. Of course, any drug that causes hallucinations (i.e., illegal drugs like cocaine, peyote, and mescaline) is likely to cause distortions in color perception.

Reactions to drugs and medications may vary. But when medications are used for chronic or life-threatening ailments, your options are limited. It may be necessary to take something that can keep a major physical problem in check, even if minor problems result. The pros and cons have to be weighed, and decisions must be made. Open discussion is necessary, and people need to have the facts.

Antibiotics. These drugs may cause loss of, or disturbance of, color vision. NegGram, often used to treat acute urinary tract infections, frequently causes blue vision confusion as well as sensitivity to light. Grisactin, an antifungal used to treat ringworm of the nails and skin, may cause a person to see as if looking through a green haze.

Barbiturates. These drugs are used for hypertension, sleeplessness, and the control of epilepsy. Use of these sedatives can result in failure to register or correctly interpret certain information, including true colors. This is usually a short-term effect, lasting perhaps hours.

Benzedrine. This drug is an amphetamine that is used as a stimulant. It can cause blue vision confusion and may sometimes cause confusion of other colors. Some people say they have seen rainbows when using this drug.

Contraceptive pills. These have been know to cause a reduction in the ability to see blue-yellow colors.

Digitalis glycosides. Sold as digoxin, this drug is used in cases of hypertension and cardiac stimulation, and may cause people to see halos. (See inset on page 62.) Digitalis usage was probably the reason that the artist Vincent van Gogh placed halos on so many objects in his paintings. He was known to consume large amounts of this substance in the form of a popular drink of the time, Absynthe, which can be very toxic. Digitalis sometimes causes everything to be seen as yellowish, or causes red-brown confusion.

Disulfiram. This drug is used in the treatment of alcoholism. It causes red-green vision disturbance.

Ethambutol hydrochloride. This drug is an anti-tubercular drug that causes red-green disturbance. Tuberculosis was, until recently, considered a disease that had been wiped out in the United States. It has, unfortunately, made a comeback.

Ariel J. was prescribed Ethambutol in high doses after being diagnosed with tuberculosis, and he is a perfect example of why an effective medication is not administered today due to side effects.

Ariel was an Israeli military prisoner of war in Syria for over two years. When he was exchanged, he was so emaciated that, at first, it was assumed that his sickly condition was due mainly to malnutrition. But then it was found that he had tuberculosis as well. So Ethambutol had to be given in high doses as his condition was critical.

At first, when Ariel noticed he had lost his color vision, it was assumed that he may be in a permanent delirious state due to malnutrition. But then it became obvious that his mind functioned fine. It was then assumed that he may have suffered a trauma to the head because he had fallen when he was shot in action. But this did not answer all the questions. Ariel also lost the capacity to distinguish grey, blue, and green as well as to distinguish between yellow and white. Moreover, he suddenly needed strong reading glasses for nearsightedness.

For a number of years, Ariel considered himself lucky to be alive. He went into denial about his permanent loss of color vision. But he now knows that one of the side effects of Ethambutol is color vision loss that can be permanent and disturbing.

Ethchlorvynol. This drug is distributed under the name Placidyl, and is a controlled substance used as a sedative and in the treatment of insomnia. It can cause red-green color vision disturbance.

Indomethacin. This drug is often used in the treatment of arthritis. Not only is it an anti-inflammatory drug, it is also an analgesic. Indomethacin may cause blue-green-yellow vision disturbance. This CVC is reversible if the patient discontinues use of the drug.

Lasix. This drug is commonly used to curb high blood pressure. It is also used to control edema (swelling caused by water-retention) and to treat certain kidney problems. Lasix sometimes causes very upsetting side effects of altered, disturbed, or defective color vision. (See *Medicine: Cure or Cause?* on page 62.) Once use of this drug is stopped, color vision should return.

Nitroglycerin. This drug is used by angina patients and can cause temporary blue-yellow vision confusion. The time periods of the effects may vary.

Thorazine, and a number of other medications that are used to treat nervous disorders and psychological problems can cause a person to see as if through a blue haze. Sometimes used to treat depression, these drugs can actually cause people to feel as "blue" as everything around them appears to be.

Again, please keep in mind that color vision is a small price to pay if your medication is keeping you alive or making your life worth living. Please consult with your physician before discontinuing use of any prescription that you may think is distorting your perception of colors.

Industrial Toxins

Many studies have shown that strong chemicals can cause color vision alterations. Synthetic chemicals are the worst offenders. The pollution they cause has been shown to be responsible for many cases of CVC that are not registered in official statistics about the condition. A study conducted in 1987 showed that chemically induced CVC can become permanent. In most cases, this type of acquired color vision confusion or loss returns when workers leave their jobs for extended periods lasting weeks. The rate at which color vision returns may vary. But it will not remain if toxins affect the eyes again.

In a recent test, which verified other tests of this nature, workers in a paint manufacturing plant were studied for differences in chemical exposure and CVC. Some, such as office workers, had little direct exposure to the chemicals while some had constant exposure. The Farnsworth-Munsell Test (see page 107) was administered to determine whether there was loss of color vision. Of those who were constantly exposed to solvents, 80 percent had color vision loss. Among those who had less contact with the solvents, 23 percent had color vision loss. All who worked in the plant were affected, and nearly 30 percent showed some permanent damage.

Workers in the petrochemical (natural gas) industries have also been found to be affected by CVC. One wonders about those who work with pesticides and pharmaceuticals.

Color vision loss that results from exposure to chemicals or solvents appears to be caused by neural rather than ocular damage. In other words, in these cases it was not the retina but the nerves that transmit visual information to the brain that are affected. This was reported in 1987 by a team from the University of Quebec.

Listed here are some of the chemicals that depress the capacity to see colors.

Carbon disulfide. This chemical has been used in the preparation of hides, to prevent mildew growth, and in the production of rayon, rubber, explosives, insecticides, and even wallpaper. Those exposed to carbon disulfide have reported red-green vision confusion and poor ability to judge just how light or dark a color is (its value and chroma). If no action is taken, blue vision is lost and finally total color vision loss occurs.

Carbon monoxide. A poisonous gas, carbon monoxide is formed by incomplete combustion of materials that contain carbon, such as gasoline. Among those affected by loss of color vision associated with this industrial toxin are bus drivers, who are continuously exposed to exhausts given off by their buses, and bus passengers who breathe this exhaust inside bus stations. Some bus drivers claim to have missed stopping at red traffic lights because of loss of sensitivity to the color red. The condition has been a problem particularly in Eastern European countries and Third World countries, where engine parts are scarce and regulations regarding proper upkeep of commercial vehicles are poorly enforced.

Recently, one of the responses to the problem in Russia has been to take away the driver's license of anyone who has red color vision confusion, whether it is inherited or acquired. This policy has led to a jump in sales of bogus drivers' licences on Russia's black market—there's no need to pass a color vision test, just have the payoff ready!

Fertilizers, bug sprays, and antifreeze. These toxins were first implicated in cases of CVC in 1971. Again, red-green color vision loss was reported.

Lead and lead-based chemicals. These chemicals are often found in storage batteries, in old plumbing, in many old paints, and gasoline. They can cause permanent red-green vision disturbance. Although the manufacture of lead-based items has declined significantly, there are still many products that are painted with lead-based paint, such as renovated antique furniture.

Styrene. A colorless oily liquid with a strong aroma, styrene is often mixed with other materials, such as rubber, because it is water-resistant, weather-resistant, scratch-resistant, and easy to clean with alcohol-based cleaning fluids. It is also very combustible. Styrene is used for making polystyrenes, plastics, and rubber. Styrene resin is used in boat-building. This widely used industrial solvent has neurotoxic effects; it attacks the optic nerve fibers and the blue-vision cones.

Research conducted in 1991 focused on seven small plastics factories in Milan, Italy. It was found that the extent of the damage caused by styrene vapors given off in the manufacturing process, or released when an item that contains styrene is burned, can depend on the amount to which a person has been exposed. But that damage can take place rather quickly if levels of styrene are high. Blue-yellow color vision disturbance was most common, but some workers were also affected by red-green vision confusion. It is possible to monitor styrene overexposure by testing the urine of employees.

Why does the government allow the use of such chemicals? The answer is simple. People like the look, convenience, and easy care of products that contain these materials. Little attention is paid to the toxic waste, the danger of loss of vision or loss of color vision. Just consider that when polystyrene burns, it releases central nervous system depressants and irritants. And, this substance is found nearly everywhere—in your home in the form of additives to washable paints, in plastic items, and in furniture coverings. You might well guess that firemen are in constant danger of color vision confusion or loss.

Other Causes of Acquired CVC

Aging. As we reach the age of sixty, some physical changes occur in our capacity to see colors. In 1991, a study was done in Canada with people aged thirty to ninety to learn how much loss of color vision occurs with age. It was found that rapid change in color vision seems to take place after the age of sixty. By the age of seventy, people seem to have a harder time differentiating between blue and purple. Although the sample of sixty-eight people was not big, the findings were significant, and it would be worthwhile to pursue the study on a larger scale.

You might wonder what the benefit is of knowing that our ability to see colors may diminish as we age. Armed with the knowledge of specific problems, we would be able to decorate and illuminate the homes of older persons in order to provide greater comfort and more independent living. Pharmaceutical firms might learn the most appropriate colors for pills that older persons tend to take. Older Americans would find it comforting to know that others are similarly affected, and that loss of color vision is a natural result of aging. Perhaps most importantly, we would be able to present printed and televised information to older adults in a clear manner.

As we age, medical conditions, including cataracts and other eye ailments, Alzheimer's, Parkinson's, and diabetes, may worsen. The accumulated effects of medication taken for a long time may begin to show. These effects may be compounded by the effects of medication being taken for newly developed medical problems. In addition, the homes of older people are often poorly lit because they worry about the cost of electricity. And an unwillingness to admit to the reality of visual changes doesn't help either.

Argon lasers. The word laser stands for Light Amplification by Stimulated Emission of Radiation. Lasers are used as cutting tools in industry and in medicine. People who use lasers on a regular basis have been shown to acquire blue-yellow color vision confusion. These people also have damaged retinas from "flashbacks" of laser beams that bounced off contact lenses.

Cigarette smoke. The exact extent of CVC from cigarette smoke and the reason are not yet quite clear because very little attention has been focused on the problem. Perhaps the damage is caused by smoke rising directly to the eye, or perhaps by some chemical in cigarettes that causes deterioration of cones or ocular nerves.

IN CONCLUSION

Unfortunately, interest in acquired CVC has been minimal. The chemical industry has not even admitted to the possibility of chemically induced color vision loss. The industry has tried to protect its "innocence" to assure that law suits will not deplete its assets. The tobacco industry has acted in the same manner, while the medical and pharmaceutical industries simply ignore the topic. And the average person is as much to blame as industry. When industrial employees are being tested for the effects of occupational hazards, few think to note their color vision, and even fewer report disturbances with it. The relatively low number of occupationally related cases of CVC does not mean that the problem doesn't exist, but that few consider it significant enough to report.

Will the incidence of acquired CVC increase in the coming years? We know that loud rock and roll music has sometimes pierced eardrums. Similarly, traffic noises, jackhammers, and other industrial noises have caused hearing loss. It may well be that the "color-screaming" today—in television presentations, in toys, in clothing— may prove to be hazardous to our sensing of delicate, elegant, and understated colors. At this time, we should learn all we can about CVC in order to prevent and/or deal with the condition.

Once people know they have CVC, they can examine the causes and possible coping techniques (see Chapter 11). Some cases of acquired color vision loss are not severe and last for only a short time. If the cause of the problem can be, and is, taken away, the condition may improve with time. If the cause is not removed, damage may become permanent. Other cases tend to be progressive in nature, getting worse with time. People whose color vision loss is caused by chronic ailments that get worse over time must assuredly learn how to cope. People who take medications that are necessary for life may have no choice but to put up with CVC as a side effect. But now that you are armed with the facts, your decisions can be made wisely and, hopefully, more easily.

6

Colorblindness in Females

You may be wondering whether there is a sufficient reason to devote an entire chapter to colorblindness in women. There certainly is. We must first put to rest the common misconception that females cannot have color vision confusion. The truth is, three out of every hundred women are born with this problem. If you consider that every male who has inherited the gene for colorblindness did so from a female, the number of females who carry the gene for colorblindness is larger still.

The number of documented cases of women who experience difficulties with color vision is forcing people to rethink their opinions. We should all be aware that although females are affected by color vision confusion in the same way as men, their problem has a different angle.

For one thing, statistics regarding inherited color vision confusion among women are even less accurate than those for men. All-encompassing research has not been conducted for either males or females, and the opportunities to gather statistics have been even fewer among women. Until recently, most jobs that required testing for color vision were not even optional for females. Women did not become construction workers, railroad engineers or conductors, commercial airplane pilots, electrical workers, etc. on a regular basis until the "sexual revolution." In addition, even when a women admits she is colorblind, few people believe her. For some reason, the notion that females cannot inherit color vision confusion seems to persist in the minds of most people.

At a 1984 computer graphics convention, a German electrical engineer told a story of exactly this kind of bias. The engineer himself is not colorblind. He knows this for sure because his engineering school required that his color vision be tested before he began his studies. Subsequently, he became an employee of an architectural firm.

When this firm became "high-tech," a whole staff of clever computer programmers was hired. Before architectural drafting was done by computer, draftsmen had to pass a color vision test. The company's new employees did not have to take such a test—after all, they have access to a powerful machine that can produce things in color at the touch of a key. They were hired because of their computer expertise, not their grasp of graphics or colors.

When a male computer programmer who was colorblind was asked to design a program with various colors, he was afraid to say he could not. He wanted to keep his well-paying job at this very exacting and prestigious firm. So, he, asked a female computer operator to help him out. She did. But she did not let on that she was colorblind, too!

The result of their collaboration was useless to the firm. After a number of presentations were thrown out, both computer operators admitted they could not handle that particular task.

The higher-ups believed the man, who said he needed to work on tasks that would not require accurate color vision. But the woman's claim was questioned. She was considered professionally unqualified and was "demoted" to clerical work. She quit.

Of course, you now know that a man who inherits the gene for colorblindness from his mother will exhibit color vision confusion, but a woman needs to inherit the gene from both her mother and father. Although there are fewer females than males who are colorblind, many women are "carriers" of the condition. It had been believed that such carriers were not hampered visually, however, recent tests, have shown that these carriers often have less color sensitivity than others. There are times when they may have some doubts about the colors they see.

As you read about the women who have inherited CVC, consider how difficult it is for any female to hold a professional position. When a colorblind woman is found wanting, she gets little sympathy and has little recourse.

IGNORANCE ISN'T BLISS

A waitress in a coffee shop in Canada was bemoaning her plight. Her mother-in-law, who was always a nice lady, and was now widowed, had moved in with her and her husband. The couple tried to cheer the widow by decorating her room in dusty pink, but all they got were complaints. The widow said that the color of the room was depressing. Not only that, she had taken to wearing outlandish colors that made her the laughingstock of the town. True, one must forgive a woman who was past seventy. But why would she say that pink is depressing? It never occurred to the waitress that her mother-in-law might not have been able to distinguish pink from blue, and blue might depress her.

The waitress recalled that her mother-in-law had actually never done any decorating herself. Her husband's strong-willed father had made all the selections in the house, even choosing his wife's wardrobe. She had always believed that since the father-in-law held the purse strings, the mother-in-law had little to say in that regard. It had never entered her mind that the mother-in-law did not decorate or select her own clothes because she was colorblind. When the waitress got a plausible explanation of the possibility that her mother-in-law may be colorblind, she felt relieved—she was not at fault.

A young woman of African-American heritage applied to the Health Sciences program at East Carolina University in 1992, only to be told she could not be accepted. She had achieved high scores in math and biology on all of her college aptitude tests, and she had applied to this particular school because she believed in its claims to be "color blind" when it came to race. At first, she wondered if she had been turned down for the program because of her heritage. As it turned out, this woman had tested as colorblind, that is color vision deficient, when she took a color vision test required for applying to that program. She had never known of her CVC because her family members all saw colors the same way she did, and they had never made any fuss over it. She had always thought that her preferences for certain colors were due to cultural differences, but they were actually due to a vision problem. Sadly, her dream of entering her local college's medical program was crushed. Had she been tested for CVC earlier in her life, and counseled for it, she may have been better prepared. It was little comfort to this woman to find out that an applicant for the dermatology program at the same school had been rejected because he could not distinguish blotches on skin.

Mind you, it was known long ago that women can inherit the condition. In 1927, Dr. George Waaler, of the University of Oslo in

Norway, reported that among the people he was testing in his research on color vision, he found women who were red-green colorblind. This was a surprise to some, particularly since there were no statistics on females with colorblindness. How could there be statistics? Waaler was the first researcher to include females in his scientific study. Women have often not been included in other research dealing with medicine, health, or biological tendencies, and therefore there could be few statistics about them until now.

Fifteen years before Waaler presented his findings, in 1911, an American geneticist named Dr. Edmond Wilson published extensive research showing that there was a strong possibility that a woman could be colorblind, and if she was, it would happen because she had inherited faulty genes from both parents, while a male needs to inherit faulty genes only from his mother to be affected by this condition.

This was a significant step forward from a previous bit of research that was done in 1881 by Professor Johann Friedrich Horner, of the University of Zurich, in Switzerland. Horner was the one who proved that males inherit CVC, from mothers and not from fathers. He was actually studying how hemophilia was inherited when he stumbled upon this information, since the pattern of inheritance seems to be the same in both conditions. But according to him, women were never colorblind, although they were carriers of this condition. He made this mistake by assuming that if hemophilia is only found in men, this would be the case with color vision confusion. (At this time it was not common for women to have hemophilia, therefore, as with colorblindness, it was assumed that they didn't have it.)

Well, by 1927, as I mentioned before, it definitely was known that this condition can affect females. But they have rarely been tested. Because of this, and the fact that the information found in these studies was not spread to the general public, people still think that women cannot be born colorblind.

One woman, named Eileen, wrote me recently begging for proof that women can be colorblind. Eileen is in her late 20s. Her own aging mother who lives in Florida cannot accept that she has given birth to a daughter who is colorblind. The most recent skirmish between mother and daughter took place when Eileen visited her mother for her birthday. The two decided to go to Disneyworld in Orlando. At one point, they parted for a while and had agreed to meet at dinnertime in a specified area. Both had maps of the grounds. When it was time to meet, Eileen was in a quandry. The map at hand seemed to show all buildings as having "the same color." (She sent along a copy of this map to me. It appears that the colors brown and red-purple were chosen, for whatever reason, to denote buildings of varied areas.) Each building had its name printed on the map in black on top of the colored geometric figure that represented it. This young woman could not read the black on top of what seemed like another black to her. When she asked some people which building was which, they tended to shy away from her, thinking she might be unstable because she had the map at hand and could read other information, but seemed to act as if she was "strange" when it came to that map. When she found her way at last, her mother was annoyed that this holiday had to be muddled up again by this careless daughter—which, of course, lent an unhappy note to the whole attempt on her part to have a pleasant mother-daughter event with her aging mother. Eileen contacted me because she needed to prove to herself she was not at fault, that her color vision problem is real and not a form of mental instability.

It also must be taken into consideration that women tend to live longer than men. For this reason, women may be more prone to colorblindness that strikes as a result of a long-term disease than men are, as in the case of diabetes. Because they live longer, they tend to be given more medication to improve their quality of life in later years. It is very likely that these women would not report their acquired color vision confusion for fear of being labeled senile.

As for the female "carriers" who transmit the genes to sons, they may, themselves, have "off" color vision, but no one seemed to give much thought to that until recently. In 1993, it was shown by researchers from the department of Experimental Psychology of Cambridge University, in Britain, that such women do seem to have an ever so slight variation of color vision, particularly when it comes it the color red.

Unfortunately, most women still are not tested for CVC. If they were, it would probably be found that most women working in factories that produce pharmaceuticals and office supplies have acquired CVC. There are still others in the military or other outdoor careers who may have acquired CVC, though they have not been tested for it. Alice Hamilton, M.D., who founded the first Occupational and Industrial Medical program in the U.S. at the Harvard Medical School, where she was a member of the faculty since 1919, had championed control of safe work environment as long ago as 1902. Dr. Hamilton had handled cases of "phossy jaw," (a condition that destroyed the jaw bones of young women working in industries that handled phosphates, like painting watch dials that glowed in the dark and brass polishing). She was instrumental in highlighting the plight of working women's occupational hazards and passing the Occupational Health and Safety Act (OSHA) through Congress in 1970. She died shortly thereafter at the age of 101. By then many young women had been on the industrial work force and could have been tested, but the possibility of acquiring color vision confusion was not recognized as a serious possibility until more recent years.

If testing for color vision were required at some occupational stage, alternatives to certain chemicals could be used, and certain safety measures could be taken in industrial settings in order to protect both women and men from acquiring CVC.

TALES FROM KINDERGARTEN

Barbara, 62, is a colorblind woman whose livelihood is jeopardized by her red-green deficiency. She was trained as a kindergarten teacher but was forced to leave her job because of the stresses associated with hiding her problem. After all, no matter how good she was as a teacher, she would be remiss if some kindergarten child failed to know the colors by the end of the year!

She tried to hide her problem by telling children not to tear the paper off the crayons. She could, thus, read the name of the crayon and be one step ahead of the unsuspecting child who might ask about it. This worked fine until she saw a child tear the paper and warned, in a panic, that she'd kill him if he ever did that again. The child returned home and complained to his mother that the kindergarten teacher threatened to kill him.

So Barbara was fired from her job and subsequently took a job as a secretary. In this line of work, she thought, she would not have to deal with colors. But the telephone on her desk had red blinkers instead of a ringer. All too often she did not answer the phone. Her employers assumed that she was frequently away from her desk or was not paying attention to her job. She tried to explain that she had a problem seeing red, but that was laughed off. How could a woman be colorblind? She was told that only men have this problem.

Now, Barbara is involved in promotional work for the mayor of a mid-sized city in upstate New York. The work primarily involves making public speaking appearances—in other words, talking. This is something she can do with great ease. But her colorblindness presents some problems even in this job. When she needed to order brochures, the matter of paper color and ink color came up. When she attended a fund-raising cocktail party, she had a hard time figuring out what food she was about to put into her mouth. Was it a black olive or a cherry tomato? Was it a grape or a green olive? Was it water or wine or what?

One can leave selection of ink and paper color to a printer, but what does one do at a fund-raiser? It's certainly not classy to sniff an appetizer or spit it out in such situations! Think about how you choose the foods you eat. Do you pick them because of colors? Have you ever even paid attention to their colors?

You do, of course, pay attention to the colors of traffic lights. To Barbara, red lights look black, the yellow resembles the color of a lemon—which she sees as light grey or white—and the green light looks orange. (Notice that even those with CVC discuss colors in terms of fruit or other common objects. It is easier for all of us to cope with and identify the vast array of colors in this manner.)

Another such tale involved a female architect who, as a child, had nearly failed kindergarten because she could not recite her colors when they were pointed out to her. For a while, she was placed among the slow students because it was assumed that a girl who was not able to distinguish colors must be slow-witted. (That this woman became an architect is not really a surprise. Many architects have color vision confusion, and therefore, are known to focus more on the effect of shadows and textures than on color use in their buildings.)

A woman who is now administrator of a university program had a similar problem in kindergarten. She was shown some cars and asked the color of each. When one particularly appealing car was held up, this student enthusiastically called out "blue" before the others could respond. The car, in fact, was purple. The child returned home feeling like a loser. Her father, a psychologist who is colorblind, listened to her tale and quickly tested her. Finding that she was clearly colorblind, he consoled her by saying that she was just like he was.

That bit of news made her very happy, but it upset her mother. The mother felt it was natural for her son to be like his father. But her daughter? Even learning that she herself obviously carried this gene could not pacify the mother. Her family had no faults, she said, and she set out to find some way to repair the "blemish" that her daughter had exhibited.

Now that the daughter is grown, she actually likes her situation. Her CVC has become an interesting conversation piece, and she has her own way of coping with it. She learned her coping skills the hard way. For instance, although she was a straight A student in her high school years, she got a "D" in a required chemistry course. Chemicals can often be recognized by color, and results of chemical reactions can be determined by resulting colors. (This was before computers were used.) Verifications of chemical reactions were made by using litmus paper, which is pink under some conditions and blue under other conditions. To her, all of these clues meant nothing. She could not determine what color she saw or what she was expected to see. The poor grade was an easy way to decide that a job involving chemicals was not her forte.

PROFESSIONAL TRIBULATIONS

Women have jumped many hurdles and made much progress as far as being considered equal to men, but when it comes to colorblindness, many women have had to go back to "square one." A young accountant recently told me about how colorblindness has affected her career and the rest of her life. It had taken her long years of study to prepare to become a CPA (certified public accountant). She had passed the same difficult exam that her male counterparts had passed. Despite her expertise in the field, she was fired from her job. It was not poor quality work that led to the firing, it was her colorblindness. The software programs used in the office were color coded, as were the files. Completed documents were placed in bins of certain colors. The woman was accused of being slow in getting started with clients and being sloppy with documents because she was forever placing them in the wrong bins. She tried to explain her problem, but her explanation was considered a "cop-out." She considered retraining for a profession in which she could avoid the pitfalls of dealing with colors. Sad to say, color coding is now being used extensively in all industries and professions. No one considers the possibility of coding materials by another system. The fault lies not with the accountant's professional skills, but with the manner in which color coding is now used.

STRANGE CASES OF COLORBLINDNESS

Being a colorblind female can make life complicated in many ways. Because society tends to believe, in general, that women are not colorblind, no testing is done, but also, as children, no coping techniques can be taught if the young girls are being told that they should be able to see colors normally. One odd case that illustrates this was written up some 40 years ago. A young girl was so overwhelmed by her inability to see colors that she eventually refused to open her eyes in school. She never played with other children and refused to go outdoors. At school, she was placed in a class for the visually impaired, which only made matters worse. Finally, she was transferred to a state school for retarded children. She was in the school for years until it was proven that she was one of the rare individuals who suffer from total colorblindness (achromatopsia). For years, no one had thought of testing her for color vision confusion.

Here's another bizarre case that was fully documented in the *Swiss Journal of Medicine* before the Second World War. One of the the first females ever recorded as being colorblind was Leonie, the daughter of a German Jewish family. Her father, who was colorblind, was a professor at a major university. Both Leonie and her twin sister had vision problems that could not be corrected by glasses.

Leonie lived her life red-green blind in her right eye, and completely blind in her left eye. She saw yellow and white as variations of light blue. The spectrum that goes from green to brown to purple to red was a total confusion for her. Her twin sister had extensive color confusion in the right eye and saw stripes with the left eye. Testing proved that the twins' mother was also colorblind.

But Leonie was not the type to be hampered by her visual problems. She was not the type to give up. During World War II, her husband had been ambushed and kidnapped by the Nazis because he was Jewish. Leonie escaped to England and, being penniless, found work at Scotland Yard, where she became a handwriting expert. Although she could not see colors properly, she could pick up the slightest variations in the shape and thickness of lines in handwriting.

A number of years ago, she wrote to tell of her experiences:

Naturally, it is very upsetting when a saleswoman does not understand the situation and entices me to buy a blue suit, an expensive purple hat and a scarf of yet another color though I detest looking like a peacock.

My sister and I have been continually trapped by our colorblindness. For instance: A life situation—are the fruits ripe and yellowed or still green? Books that have instructions or units of focus written in red are totally lost to me. There have been science texts which had red underlining or red headlines or red-colored focus paragraphs which disappeared in my sight, and yet, I could hardly explain to anyone that I could not see [the red words] if I proved to be rational and able to read the rest of the material. My sister was so disgusted that she never married, knowing full well she might cause someone else [her offspring] to be cursed. I could not resist my suitor, so I was married. [Leonie's granddaughters were not born colorblind but her grandson was].·

Leoni and her twin both lived to be 90.

IN CONCLUSION

Time and again, women have voiced their quandry: should they admit to having inherited color vision confusion and risk being considered dishonest or cop-out artists? This, of course, is not a problem faced by males who have CVC. And considering how hard it is for a woman to be accepted into certain professions in the first place, colorblind women have a particularly difficult row to hoe.

Then there are the women who are "carriers." Many silently cope with guilt, feeling that they have brought grief to their children or grandchildren. It is far more rare for colorblind men to worry about the genetic implications.

Whether in the workplace or on the home front, a woman who has color vision confusion is at a much greater disadvantage than a man. Of course, colorblind men and women both encounter many daily problems to which they must learn to adjust.

7

A Journey Through Color Vision Research

In order to attain the heights of knowledge, a sage once said, you have to stand on the shoulders of giants. In our search to understand color vision confusion, there are many shoulders upon which we can stand. However, even though colorblindness has been around since biblical times, no ancients, it seems, asked questions about the condition—at least, no record of such pondering exists. The climb to knowledge has been slow, but giants have appeared now and then, beginning with the genius Leonardo Da Vinci.

THE FIRST CLUES ABOUT COLORBLINDNESS

As with most discoveries, information about how color vision works—and therefore about colorblindness—evolved for a completely different reason. As you read in the previous chapter, the hereditary pattern of colorblindness was discovered coincidentally by a doctor studying the hereditary pattern of hemophilia. As you will read in the following pages, the study of color vision began for much more practical reasons.

Da Vinci

Leonardo da Vinci was born in Italy in 1452. Most people know him for his "Mona Lisa," but he was also an inventor and a scholar interested in the functioning of the human body and mind. Among da Vinci's inventions were military weapons. Because weapons at the time had to be aimed by eye onto the projected target in the far distance, da Vinci was interested in the various ways that people see the sky and how their vision might be distorted in fog, at sundown, and so forth. Among his observations was the notation that blue and yellow are somehow opposites. He was right. In fact, it explains why people who have a problem distinguishing blue also have a problem with yellow.

Tuberville

Some two hundred years later, in 1684, an account was published about "Several Remarkable Cases in Physick Relating Chiefly to the Eyes," by D. Tuberville in the Philosophical Transaction of the Royal Society of London. He pointed out that some healthy people seemed to have odd color vision.

Huddart

Nearly one hundred years passed before another account of color-blindness appeared in literature. In 1777, "Of a Person Which Could Not Distinguish Colors" also appeared in the Royal Society of London's journal. This report by J. Huddart told of a shoemaker named Harris who could not pair brown and black shoes properly. The clever man took in black shoes on Mondays, Wednesdays, and Fridays and brown shoes on the other three days of the week.

In 1778, the same journal carried a report entitled, "An Account of a Remarkable Imperfection of Sight." But it was not until 1794 that solid scientific examination of colorblindness condition was published. At that time, John Dalton of Manchester, England, opened the door to understanding the extent of what happens in the daily life of someone who has color vision confusion.

Dalton

John Dalton, who was colorblind, was a British physicist and mathematician. He had wanted to be a botanist until he was told that the geraniums he thought were blue were actually seen as pink by others. He did not have a university education. No college would admit him; they thought he was dim-witted. Because he was unable to distinguish the colors of chemicals, he could not study the chemistry required at British universities. Yet Dalton developed the atomic theory upon which the atomic chart, familiar to anyone who studies chemistry, is based. His theory enabled industry to develop chemical formulas and to be certain of the outcome of mixing specific amounts of chemicals. Had it not been for Dalton's contribution to the world of science, metallurgy, large-scale food processing, and the pharmaceutical industries as well as the textile industry could not produce consistent-looking items that have the same properties.

Dalton is also recognized as the father of meteorology, although he never did see the colors in the aurora borealis or in lightning, whose electric output he studied. Nor did he ever see the colors of a rainbow. He wrote a book on meteorology in which he used the word "rainbow," but only to refer to its shape, not to its colors.

After he published that book, titled *Meteorological Observations and Essays* in 1793 at the age of twenty-seven, he was invited to join the Manchester Literary and Philosophical Society. Given the opportunity to address the group the following year, he decided to speak about his findings regarding the odd color vision he and his brother experienced. He called his presentation "Extraordinary Facts Relating to the Vision of Colors: With Observations by Mr. John Dalton."

The stunning revelation of the talk—the details that he had collected and presented as if he and his brother were scientific specimens to be studied—were a sensation. Dalton told the society's members:

> I see only two or three distinctions [in colors]. This should call yellow and blue, or yellow, blue and purple.
>
> My yellow comprehends the red, orange, yellow and green of others; and my blue and purples coincide with theirs."

He said, in effect, that red and green appeared the same to him—a yellow orange—but what kind of yellow-orange did he see? We will never know.

In 1836, Dalton was honored with a doctorate from Oxford University. For this, his first university degree, it is said, he "seemed to make a fool of himself." He proudly appeared at that important event wearing a crimson colored cape, which he ordered from a tailor after selecting the material himself. Under other conditions, he would not wear loud colors because it was unbecoming to his Quaker faith. On this occasion he was happy to state honestly that to him, the red looked black.

Goethe

In 1810, the German poet and playwright Johann Wolfgang von Goethe published a book entitled *Farbenlehre,* or *color study* in German. Goethe had long studied the effects of colors on vision. He wanted to know whether people who have normal color vision can have their vision distorted for the purpose of creating moods on the theater stage.

During his research, Goethe noted that there are people who always have distorted color vision. He referred to them as being colorblind (or *farbenblind* in German). Goethe also noted that people with normal color vision often can continue to "see" colors after there is no color to be seen because their minds carry the imagery for a while. Goethe established the significant role of the mind in relation to seeing or not seeing colors. Because Goethe was not a scientist, few took note of his ideas regarding color vision.

Just a decade after Goethe's book appeared, cases of people with odd color vision were being reported in Scotland and in the United States. In one case, a man was reported to be "insensible" to colors; in another instance, a man was said to be incapable of distinguishing colors.

The question as to whether colorblind people are blind to red raged on at the time. It was an important question. The railroads were being built, steamships began to ply the waters of the world, and steam was being introduced as a form of power in industry. All of these required that the steam in the boilers be monitored; workers had to check gauges on which information was printed in black and red. Red colored information warned of potentially dangerous developments.

Seebeck

In 1837, the question of who saw red was solved when a German scientist named Albrecht Seebeck proved that some of those who have red vision confusion do not see red at all, but that most see it in one form or another. His observations, like those of Dalton, needed refining by others later on, but he did make a valid point at a crucial time.

Young

Some of the refining was done by an English physician named Thomas Young. Young developed the wave theory of light and postulated a three-color theory of color vision. An amateur musician, Young believed that light, like sound, must function in waves. He measured light waves of different colors and theorized that the retina must contain sensors that can respond to the different lengths of light.

Young theorized that those who have red colorblindness may have an absence or a paralysis of the "fibers" of the retina that normally cause a person to see red. He had no idea what these fibers would look like, but he sensed they were there. Dalton had chided Young for his theories and decided to leave his eyes to science at his death to prove Young wrong. When Dalton died in 1844, his eyes were dissected by Dr. George Wilson in the presence of Dr. David Brewster. Also colorblind, Brewster was then editor of the *Edinburgh Journal of Medicine*. (Brewster's fortune was made when he invented the kaleidoscope which became a favorite toy of Queen Victoria, who knighted him.) In dissecting the eyes, Wilson found nothing unusual—of course, the electron microscope had not yet been invented, nor was electricity. Wilson went on to publish his findings in 1857 in a book titled *Researches in Color Blindness*, in which he included a warning about hiring colorblind people for maritime and railroad work.

Because of Dalton's role in the study of colorblindness, the condition became known as "Daltonism." To this day, it is called by that name in some languages. It has even been referred to as "Dalton Mania" although, clearly, Dalton was not a maniac nor are others who have the condition. After Dr. Wilson's book was published, the name for the condition he used in his title became the accepted name in English. From then on, the condition was called "colorblindness."

Helmholtz

One modern theory of color vision is known as the Young-Helmholtz theory. It was introduced in 1852 by a German physiologist named Hermann von Helmholtz, who, like Young, thought that there are three color receptors in the retina. These are sensitive to either short, medium, or long range light waves, but when they are stimulated together, they produce the sensation of the colors red, green, and blue.

Helmholtz felt that it would be rare for none of the receptors to be stimulated at any one time. In fact, his idea was that each was stimulated to varying degrees at all times, thus enabling us to see a varied selection of colors. Eager to find these receptors, Helmholtz built a device that would allow a person to peer into another person's eye. He called it an *augen-speigel*, which in German means *eye mirror*. A primitive version of what we now know as an ophthalmoscope, the device was introduced to the scientific community in 1850 and within ten years had caused a revolution in the study of vision. The device enabled a researcher to see the blood vessels across the retina, the very section of the eye that is responsible for color vision. It helped uncover the path by which the retina converts light to electricity and sends it on to the brain, but it did not solve the question of colorblindness.

Maxwell

In 1855, a Scottish physicist named James Clerk Maxwell, who worked along with Helmholtz, postulated a theory of how you can pinpoint the various sub-colors that are not seen well by the colorblind. He spoke of the "Maxwell Triangle." Using the idea of the three receptors as the three points of this triangle, he said that if you can find the two colors that a colorblind person thinks are the same, and draw a line from one to the other and then draw a line from the third to the others, whatever colors seen on any other lines that meet where these two lines cross will also be colors that the person does not see. This made Helmholtz a super giant in the world of optics.

Hering

But someone dared to contradict Helmholtz, and his daring cost him a professional career in optics, and even today he is rarely mentioned in encyclopedias.

This man's name was Ewald Hering. He was a medical doctor who specialized in physiology. He said that in his many studies he found that red, green, and blue were not three opposite points of colors, but that yellow is somehow on the other end of the blue wave, green is somehow on the end of the red wave, and that at times when yellow and blue are in motion you see them as a twinkling white. His research also showed that people who have difficulty seeing red also often have a problem seeing green, and people who have difficulty seeing blue also have a problem seeing yellow. These findings contradicted those of Helmholtz. Hering thought that the electrical impulses in the brain often lead to results we might not expect. At that time there was no way to measure these impulses, but he was sure they could probably be measured and studied in the future. Hering published his first findings regarding color vision in 1872, and promptly became persona non grata in the world of optical research. Before this, he had threatened the credibility of Helmholtz's research when he claimed that the two eyes work together to focus on an object, while Helmholtz held that each eye focuses independently. This new finding was more than Helmholtz would allow, and he personally persecuted Hering, assuring him that he would find it difficult to find work in the field of optics.

As a result, Hering was "banished" from researching or teaching at German universities under pressure from Helmholtz. He eventually found work in Vienna and in Prague in the "East German" world, the "lesser" world in the opinion of proper Germans more than 100 years ago.

Still, Hering continued to research the mechanics of color vision, but he published on other topics. He became known for his research on the relationship between the activity of the heart and the lungs. He was also respected for his research on the physiology of blood cells. In fact, Hering became a major figure in the study of physiology, but he did not publish on optics until Helmholtz died.

Only in 1905 did Hering publish on optics again. He was then past sixty years of age. By then, the theories of Helmholtz were assumed to be facts, and the world of optics still did not pay attention to Hering. But things were about to change. By the turn of the century, revolutionary research in various fields of study was being conducted that would dramatically change the way people saw themselves and their world. For instance, the study of the workings of the brain was advancing, while the field of psychology was booming, particularly in Vienna where Sigmund Freud worked.

Hering's findings were of great interest to the early psychologists who focused on how the mind and eye interact, how the mind affects what we see, and how we perceive what we see and what we have mentally recorded. Hering's findings were also of interest to those in the fledgling world of advertising, which was looking to figure out the eye-mind connection and how to sway consumers' desires.

Hering himself had always been very careful about making sure he was not seen as one who had faith in crystals or read meaning into the auras of colors. He dealt with facts. He dealt with that which had been proven in experiments time and time again. He dealt with statistics. He dealt with science. He did not want to be lumped in with the likes of people who claimed that they could gauge the intelligence of a person by counting the bumps on his head. Yes, there were such people in the middle of the 19th century who espoused the pseudoscience of phrenology and actually believed that the capacity for color vision was located in the eyebrows! This may sound like nonsense to us today, but a phrenological explanation of color vision sounded much more convincing than what scientists were saying in the 19th century—that vision is produced in the back of the head even though the eyes are in the front of the head.

Piotrowski

Still, between the 1860s and the end of the 1880s, many parts of the color vision puzzle were uncovered. In 1868, a professor named Piotrowski from the Polish University of Krakow presented a person who could see only in grey tones, unable to see any colors. This condition is now called achromatopsia. It appears to be the first reported scientific case of this type of colorblindness.

Horner

In 1878, Johann Friedrich Horner, a Swiss neurosurgeon, proved that males inherit colorblindness from females. Horner's work validated the beliefs of a physician named Christian Friedrich Nasse who, in 1820, had postulated but had not proven that colorblindness is inherited through a sex gene. Horner proved that women inherit the gene for colorblindness from their fathers and transmit it to their sons, not unlike the path taken by the gene for hemophilia. Horner, however, failed to recognize the possibility of colorblindness in females. He said that no female could be colorblind, although Dalton had suggested that females may be born colorblind.

Rood

In 1879, a professor of art from Massachusetts named Ogden Rood published a book titled *Modern Chromatics*. In this book, Rood stated that a person does not see a color in isolation. A person's ability to see a color is affected by nearby colors. Nothing exists in our vision without something with which to contrast it. In effect, Rood expanded on Hering's findings.

In regard to those who have color vision confusion, Rood wrote:

It not unfrequently happens that persons with this defect remain for years unconscious of it. In one remarkable instance a bystander, in attempting to help a colour-blind person who was under investigation, showed that he was himself colour-blind, but belonged to another class!

The artist James MacNeil Whistler, who was then in Europe studying how grey, black, and white in light and shadow can be used to create visual compositions, was fascinated with Rood's book and told everyone he could about it. These two American-born men planted the seeds of what grew to be French Post-impressionism, although Rood did not like the paintings that were based on his book one bit. Still, people who have color vision confusion tend to delight in these paintings, as if they were made just for them, particularly the works of George Seurat, who seems to have used Rood's book like a recipe book for creating colored area perceptions.

Konig

In 1887, a German psychophysicist, Arthur Konig, who was a former student of Helmholtz, presented the first case of blue color vision confusion. It turned out to be due to an illness. (An inherited blue colorblindness was only verified years later.) The excitement in the medical world was great. In a period of thirty years, more information about color vision confusion was uncovered than in all the centuries before combined.

DEVELOPING THE TESTS

It was only natural that with all of these discoveries being made about colorblindness, researchers would want to know who was actually colorblind. Industry was also itching to get its hands on a test that could be used for potential employees who needed to have color vision; and the military, of course would want to test for colorblindness. But could you test for it?

Ever since steam power was used in industry, more and more concerns were being voiced about the possibility that industrial accidents were being caused by colorblind workers. This was assumed because gauges and various signals relied on the color red to denote danger.

As railways expanded and shipping increased, industry extended its use of chemicals and of steam power to run machinery. Hot air balloons were being sent up to the heavens, and there was a rumor about the coming of a horseless carriage, which, no one doubted, would run amuck. Reports of accidents increased. Industrialists and insurance companies sought protection from the causes. But there was no system for detecting whether a worker was colorblind. Once again, some suggested that physical features might be a clue. Could you tell whether someone was colorblind by the flatness of the skull just below the eyebrows, for instance?

Strutt's Test

John William Strutt, an English physicist and mathematician, demonstrated that there are people who cannot see green. He showed that there are two groups of people who have green confusion: those who say that yellow appears reddish to them, and those who say that yellow is greenish. He postulated that this color confusion happens due to heredity. Eventually, Strutt became Lord Rayleigh after he was knighted by Queen Victoria for his invention of the anomaloscope, a device used in the detection of colorblindness even today.

Strutt also had much to do with the discovery that there are some people who do not see blue properly. He noted this when he studied the various blues of the sky. He then became interested in the blue color of gas flame, and he became aware that some do not see the variations of the blues of the sky or the gas flame. Strutt's studies on how and when the blue colors of the sky become distorted or change or are confused by some were considered so important to the United States Air Force many years later, that it bought his papers which are now housed in the Rayleigh Archives at the Cambridge Research Lab in Bedford, Massachusetts.

Stilling's Test

Actually, a reliable test for colorblindness had been designed in 1876 by Jakob Stilling. The test consisted of dots of colors of varying intensities that comprised particular designs. The designs were clear to people who had full color vision, but were not seen by those who were colorblind. Stilling's test was largely ignored.

Holmgren's Test

In 1878, a test designed by a Swedish doctor named Freidrich Holmgren became the accepted test for colorblindness. The test consisted of 3 large skeins of wool, each of a different color, and 125 small wool samples dyed to various hues and various saturations of color and lightness. One of the big skeins would be thrown out for a person to see. The person would then have to find 6 or 8 wool samples that appeared to be in the same family. When that was finished, the test was repeated with the second big skein and then the third.

The test sometimes seemed to go on forever. And then the wool would get dirty with handling or carelessness, or it might be left out in the sun and the colors would fade. Eventually, the test was abandoned because half of those who should have been detected as colorblind were not, and many who had no color vision problems became nervous wrecks at the thought of taking the test and managed to fail it.

But at least a test had been devised. And there was a rush to give the test, especially after the renowned Dr. Benjamin J. Jeffries gave a lecture in Boston in 1879 on the dangers and need for detection of colorblindness. This sounded like a call to action.

Widespread Testing

Tests were soon given to children in the Boston school system and to railroad workers in the United States, France, India, England, and Germany. Employees of the Royal Cheese factory in Saltzburg, Austria, were also tested,94
as were recruits into the United States military.

The United States Army had a particularly interesting reason for wanting a test. Approximately fifteen years had passed since the end of the Civil War. As emotions cooled and reasonable people began to study what had transpired, it was determined that in the war between the Blue and Grey, many dead and wounded had been shot by soldiers on their own side. Apparently, even the Southern General Stonewall Jackson had been shot by mistake by his own troops. Obviously, there were many recruits who could not tell blue from grey. Some never saw the red flares of warning that had been sent up at night. And some could not follow the colors of their respective battalion flags because they could not see them, especially in bad weather.

Also, the U.S. Navy and Marines were beginning to play an ever-growing role in international waters, which now had color-coded rules of the sea.

THE COLORBLINDNESS BIAS

By the end of 1879, the Army began checking recruits for colorblindness. The Surgeon General of the United States suggested to President Chester Arthur that the requirement for such testing become a law of the United States Congress. Senator Benjamin Harris of Massachusetts introduced the bill in 1881 and President Arthur sent a message to

Congress in December of 1883 asking for a joint resolution of Congress. No recruits could be colorblind from then on.

Soon legislation was passed in places such as Hartford, Connecticut, and other industrial cities. The laws, in effect, outlawed the hiring of men who were colorblind. Men who were shown to be colorblind could not get railway, maritime, or other jobs. Colorblindness became a cause of unemployment and a curse for the family of the person who had it.

At this time, industries were using poisonous chemicals to create colors. Names of colors used in the computer graphics field today—cyan for blue and magenta for red—come from the names of the chemicals that were used in those days to make the colors. But the chemical magenta has long been banned because it was shown to poison printers as early as 1866, although its use continued for some time. Cyan was made from cyanide, which was proven to be poisonous as well. People from Australia to Paris were being poisoned by wearing green socks dyed with Sheele's green, which was made with arsenic. Copper oxide fumes from green made from arsenic were said to seep from wallpaper, poisoning whole families in their fancy dining rooms in Berlin. Lead and other poisons were found in paints used to color children's toys and clothing. Luckily, no one could blame the colorblind for all of this. Some even began to suspect industrial poisoning as a cause of acquired color vision loss in workers.

As if laws against hiring colorblind men for certain jobs were not enough to keep these men from earning good wages, a book titled *Heads and Faces and How to Study Them* appeared in 1892 to marginalize them even more. This book was published in New York by a company headed by Charlotte Fowler Wells, who listed herself as a pioneer of phrenology. Specifically, this book advised women to avoid marrying colorblind men to avoid going hungry or being shamed out of good social graces.

This book became a best seller, and one hundred thousand copies were sold. It offered a do-it-yourself method for determining colorblindness. The capacity for colorblindness, the book stated, is located on the brow, almost directly over the eyeball. In those with upward and forward arching brows, you can be sure that they have very fine color vision. In fact, the book stated that a man with such eyebrows can stand at one end of a path in the park and see twenty-five or thirty shades of green under the eye at once. Heaven help anyone who did not have the right arch in the eyebrows!

With so much going against colorblind men, it is not surprising that when it became known that the United States Army would take anyone as a foot soldier to fight the war in Europe in 1914, many were willing to go. By the end of that war, it had become evident that colorblind men are often far better sharpshooters than others. The Germans had introduced a new military color that they called *feldsgrau* or *field-grey*, today known as khaki. They said it was a form of protection for the soldier in the field, and they even added camouflage. The Germans did not know that the United States had dropped its ban on colorblind soldiers, and it was proven that the colorblind troops could spot movements others could not. As a result, colorblind soldiers popped the pointed helmets off the Kaiser's men without being fooled by camouflage as others might have been.

As industry developed after World War I, it was clear that a better test for color vision had to be found, and that it had to be administered without the hysteria of the previous era.

Munsell's Color System

Alfred Munsell, an American from Boston, had been studying art in Paris when Impressionism began to bloom. He returned to Boston, became an art instructor at a teacher's college, and, within a few years, created the wheel that carries his name to this day—the Munsell Color Wheel. While Goethe and da Vinci said that blue is the opposite of yellow, Munsell called yellow and blue primary colors along with red. Opposite blue, he placed orange and opposite yellow, he placed violet. Opposite red, he placed green.

Munsell copied his ideas from a color wheel created by the French chemist M.E. Chevreul in 1839. Chevreul was, at the time, the director of dyes at the Manufactures Royales De Goblin, the national tapestry workshop of France. But Chevreul got the idea from Morris Harris, who produced the first color wheel in 1766 in England, where he was an entomologist. Morris needed to specify the colors of the insects he was studying, and wanted to create a standard of color for naturalists.

Munsell called orange, violet, and green secondary colors. What is a secondary color? According to Munsell, the secondary colors are produced by mixing two of the primary colors together, but a primary color cannot be mixed from anything. (This is true if you deal with paints, not light.)

Although Munsell did not speak of color vision confusion, he, in effect, actually pointed out the colors that are problems for people who have color vision confusion. Those who have a problem seeing red also tend to have a problem seeing green. Blue and orange are the colors most readily seen by those with color vision confusion while yellow and violet are relatively tricky for them.

Basically the Munsell System deals with what Munsell called the three aspects of colors: hue (color), chroma (saturation and sheen, or vibrance), and value (relative lightness or darkness). He pointed out that in some cases, a person may see the hue clearly, but may be totally thrown off by the chroma or value. Munsell showed that even those who have colorblindness can distinguish chroma, if not hue, or value if not chroma. He also showed that there can be situations where the hue is seen but the chroma or value may be "misread."

Munsell offered his color wheel to industry in 1914 as World War I was beginning. No one was particularly interested. Munsell died nearly broke in 1918 as the war ended and the influenza epidemic swept away so many. His son, however, pressed for publication, and in 1921 the Strathmore Paper Company decided to print the Munsell Color Wheel.

As soon as the color wheel was published, many uses were found. The first client for this color system was the United States Soil Conservation Service. As farming in America became more industrialized, it was necessary for farmers to determine which fertilizers to use. The idea was to match different colors of soil and plant samples against a chart to determine the need for fertilizer or other chemical additives.

The Ishihara Test

In 1924, a new test for color vision was introduced by Dr. Shinobu Ishihara, a professor of ophthalmology at Tokyo University. He had begun his work on this test while he was an instructor at the Imperial Military Medical College. The test was similar to Stilling's test, but it incorporated more delicate variations of color and intensities, as developed by Munsell's system. The test was first distributed in the United States by the Meyerowitz Company of New York City, manufacturers of dental instruments. The first company to produce instruments with color-coded marks, Meyerowitz chose an orange dot to be placed on the most commonly used instrument, as orange is seen as well by colorblind persons as those with full color vision. It was lucky that the test was printed up carefully in the United States, because the original plates of the test were destroyed in an earthquake that hit Japan in 1923.

Ishihara's test became the preferred one to use. This test showed that there were some people who had serious color vision confusion, and others whose cases were milder.

COLORS AND GESTALT PSYCHOLOGY

Germany lost the First World War, but it did not lose its position as the outstanding producer of synthetic color dyes. When the war ended, there was a tremendous market for such dyes.

Industries all over the world were using colors to enhance their products, some of which the public had never heard of before and never even thought of needing or wanting, such as electric products, housewares, tools, toys, prepared foods, chewing gum, cars, electric toy trains, and cleansers. People were goaded by advertisements to buy more, to dream of acquiring more, and to use more.

Paris had been the center of art and culture in the 19th century, but by the end of World War I, Berlin became the major center of art and culture. Even the biologist George Wald, who had been a professor at Harvard and had discovered in 1917 the importance of vitamin A to correct vision, was enticed to work in the color production industry in Berlin. There, in 1933, Wald discovered what causes the retina to see colors, and what causes some to have a lesser capacity to see colors. Goethe's observations on colors were revived. Hering got a new hearing and an opportunity at last to have his life-long research published.

In German, the word *gestalt* means totality of seeing or perception. Goethe used this word often in his book *Farbenlehre*. Gestalt psychology added to our understanding of how we make sense of what we see. Unlike the work of Freud or Jung, who focused on how the mind affects the body and how human relationships and memories are affected by the mind, Gestalt researchers wanted to know how it is that we make sense of visual information, and how we can be tricked by our eyes as well.

It all started in the 1920s when a man named Max Werthheimer was on his way to join a number of others to study visual psychology in Berlin. While sitting on the train that brought him to Germany from Austria, he watched the electric poles that passed by his window. He wondered why he "knew" that the poles remained the same size, even though he saw them get bigger as they got closer and smaller as the train moved away. It became clear to him that there was more to visual perception than what we see—there was a bigger totality to how we make mental sense of visual information. The group that was founded to research this finding decided to use Goethe's word for this occurence—gestalt.

All of the members of the Gestalt psychology group were against Adolf Hitler. When Hitler took charge of Germany in the 1930s, he made their lives unbearable and forced them to leave. But he kept their findings and used them in the most negative way against them and others. Some of the psychology researchers left for the United States, some for Israel, and some to Scandinavia.

In fact, the whole world seemed to have been on the move. The world-wide depression and the rise of dictators in the 1930s led to even more mixing of languages and cultures as people relocated.

What was needed was a practical non-linguistic way to transmit information to people quickly; visual information that was clear, that transcended language and culture, and "spoke" to everyone. And it had to stimulate the minds of those who may not see colors properly.

Birren

That was when Faber Birren found a future. Birren was an expert in the field of visual communication who was forced to drop out of the University of Chicago due to lack of funds during the Depression. He was a graduate of the Art Institute of Chicago and had studied in Paris and Berlin. While Gestalt psychology dealt with perceptions, Birren dealt with clear and exact nonverbal information, designs that would trigger a powerful message. Birren was an expert with the type of symbols that can tell you when to merge in traffic or where the men's room is no matter what language you speak. His career began when he devised symbols for use in factories in the United States. Later, the United States government asked him for suggestions on communicating with a quickly recruited, semiliterate military force made up of people from varied backgrounds. Birren's suggestions were implemented with excellent results.

In designing his symbols, Birren stressed variations of lights and textures. He emphasized the use of lines, simple bold images, and definite constant colors that would stand for something no one could question. This is of great value for those who have normal color vision as well as for those who do not.

Encouraged by what Birren had done, and by observations made at the Optical Society of America in 1943, the United States Office of Naval Research in association with Columbia University funded research in 1943 for a test for colorblindness that would replace the test designed by the Japanese. The Ishihara Test took too long and was far more intricate than the needs of the United States military.

The ensuing test was developed in conjunction with the Inter Society Color Council Subcommittee on Colorblindness. Research was conducted by Le Grand Hardy, M.D., Gertrude Rand, Ph.D., and Catherine Ritter, a nurse, at the Knapp Memorial Laboratory of Physiological Optics, of Presbyterian Hospital and the Department of Ophthalmology of the College of Physicians and Surgeons of Columbia University, in New York City. The test was called the AO/H.R.R. Pseudoisochromatic Plates Test. To this day, it is the most extensively used test for colorblindness. Some people refer to it as "the dot test."

MORE RESEARCHERS

Following World War II, strides were made in many fields of medicine, but color vision confusion was not a subject of burning interest. However, there was a need to recognize that color vision problems in industry remained. This need was recognized by various organizations. The Optical Society of America held a conference as early as 1943 in New York City at which Deanne Judd, of the National Bureau of Standards in Washington D.C., presented an overview of the problem. Now, efforts to standardize color names, their intensities and their values were needed. In 1966, the Association International De Colour (AIC) met to set some standards and make sense of color names used in industry.

Zeltzer

A few medical practitioners turned their attention to developing aids for use by those who have color vision confusion. In 1974, a Massachusetts optometrist named Dr. Harry I. Zeltzer introduced a red contact lens, which he called X Chrom. Worn only in one eye, it was meant to clarify red vision confusion. It has been used by many, even those who are not colorblind, particularly card sharks in gambling casinos who can spot marked cards more easily when wearing the lens. But the lens only enhances the sight in one eye and is best used for short periods of time only.

Dr. Zeltzer's work was based, in part, on the writings of Ogden Rood. One hundred years ago, Rood noted that persons who are colorblind to red can help themselves by looking through red glass. He noted that red glass will cause green objects to appear darker, but will not affect the luminosity of reddish objects. In contrast, if one looks through green glass, red objects will be seen—even by colorblind people—as much darker than the green because green glass does not allow the red wavelength to pass through.

Land

By the time that Zeltzer's lens appeared, Edwin Land had already rattled the world of optics with his claims and his inventions. Land invented polarized sunglasses and the Polaroid Land camera, which produced images almost instantaneously and magically.

In the 1960s Land startled the scientific community by saying that the previously held beliefs about color mixing do not explain, but rather conceal, the basic laws of color vision. Not only did his cameras make black and white photos by using red and green lenses, but he made it clear that specialists in color vision were badly off track in regard to the essentials of color perception. He claimed that as long as a scene includes two colors of varying wavelengths, the brain processes the information in two segments: one for the longer wavelength band and one for the shorter wavelength band. He did not claim to know how the brain does this, but he did conduct experiments proving that his theories were valid. His Polaroid camera works on principles others had once laughed at!

Like Ewald Hering and Ogden Rood, Land pointed out that color cues are only one aspect of visual perception. Those who do not see all visual cues—such as those with CVC—may be able to compensate through "color adaption" as Land called it in his Retinex Theory. Even those who have full color vision sometimes resort to this adaptation, as well, without realizing it.

Color confusion, Land said, can happen to the best of us. His unusual camera, which was created with information that was previously viewed as "wrong," spurred the reprinting of old texts that were long ignored. M.I.T. Press, for instance, reprinted Goethe's *Color Study*, which had been translated into English as long ago as 1840. The Harvard University Press produced Ewald Hering's *Outlines of a*

Theory of Light and Sense. It was translated from the German by Leo Hurwich, Ph.D. and Dorothea Jameson, Ph.D., a team of psychologists who had long found Hering worthy of consideration. (Both were employed by Eastman Kodak for many years. They had researched and published extensively on various aspects of vision, particularly on color vision and confusion of colors. Later, they transferred to continue their work at the Department of Psychology at the University of Pennsylvania.) Anything that could shed new light on color vision, seeing in motion, confusing colors, seeing light and colors, and even the various volumes of phrenology, was reprinted for reexamination. Gestalt had then become known as the name of a form of holistic therapy. But the works of Gestalt psychologists were already available in English ever since Kurt Koffka, one of the original Berlin group, wrote *Principles of Gestalt Psychology,* in 1935 after settling in as professor at Smith College.

Personal computers first came on the scene in 1977, and gave the public the opportunity to create color graphics simply by pressing some typewriter-like keys. This opened the door to the expanded use of color coding in business and the almost universal use of inexpensive color printing. Materials printed in color are no longer being produced only by trained artists. Never before had people who had limited experience with using colors inherited such power to use color. Now, many executives and other decision makers have to deal with color as a source of information. But few would admit to their color vision confusion. Questions regarding appropriate use of color came to the fore, but few paid attention.

Faber Birren, who by then was well-known in the field of symbolic visual communication, was concerned that virtually anyone could publish colored materials with desk-top publishing, and that others would be expected to use the information in those materials. Shortly before he died in 1984, Birren gave a lecture in which he warned of using color like some throw-away item. But those who rode high in the computer world thought they had done something nifty and had liberated everyone to do his own thing.

The computer industry began to take note that the public did not dash out to buy the color-producing invention. That was when I was invited to speak at computer graphics conferences. The first major invitation came when the Canadian government added a minister of computer technologies to the cabinet. A conference titled COMPINT was held in 1985 in Montreal. People who could provide insight to the problem of communication via computer graphics were invited to offer their input. I spoke on color miscommunication. People in the computer graphics industry began to warn that more attention be paid to the proliferation of color use. They began to recognize that there might be very costly consequences due to confusion of visual information which is presented in poorly selected color codes and charts. One of the more recent findings is that focusing too long on computer monitors may be a cause of color vision confusion. But, it is also a fact that if it were not for advances in technology, we would not have graphic images of microscopic things and other such wonders.

Verriest

It has also become apparent that people can acquire colorblindness for a number of reasons (see Chapter 5). A major force in uncovering the medical and industrial causes of colorblindness was the Belgian physician Guy Verriest. Early in his career, Verriest found that color vision confusion or loss of color vision can be due to alcoholism, or at least to cirrhosis of the liver, which often develops in long-term alcoholics.

In 1964, Verriest reported that with cirrhosis of the liver, vitamin A cannot be delivered to the eyes. The retinas are, in effect, starved of a basic nutrient. Verriest felt that self-inflicted alcohol pollution was bad, but industrial pollution, which the average person cannot control, was even worse. After all, what people inflict on themselves may be their choice and they can take steps to do something about it, but industrial pollution is foisted on everybody, even people who try to live rational, healthful lives.

Although the United States National Standards Bureau was aware of increasing pollution as early as 1944, no one gave it much thought because industrial expansion was then considered more important than the "small" side effects. When industrial production expanded after World War II, various synthetics that had never existed before became abundant. All sorts of pollutants filled the air, and waste toxins were dumped in lakes, rivers, and oceans. This has affected the waters and atmosphere all over the world. Verriest considered the matter important enough to convene a world conference and to lead a significant effort to develop awareness of, and find solutions for, the harm of industrial pollution.

The first conference of the organization that he formed, the International Research Group on Color Vision, was held at Ghent in 1971.

Among the core group that attended this gathering was an outstanding team of researchers from the University of Chicago, Joel Pokorny, Ph.D., and Vivianne C. Smith, Ph.D.

These two researchers have made many discoveries regarding color vision disturbances, both inherited and acquired. Along with Verriest they coauthored the first major reference on the subject of color vision loss due to industrial pollution. The book was published in 1979.

Verriest himself was a candidate for colorblindness because he had a lifelong case of diabetes. He died suddenly of a heart attack on the way to a conference in Australia in 1988, but his work is being continued by others.

Nathans

As researchers continue trying to solve the puzzle of what leads us to inherit color vision or color vision distortions, amazing scientific discoveries are made. One of the most exciting recent discoveries came in 1988 when the genes for human color vision were located by a team headed by Jeremy Nathans, M.D., Ph.D., of the Department of Molecular Biology and Genetics of the Howard Hughes Medical Institute at John Hopkins University School of Medicine in Maryland. Genes were found to be located on the upper right arm of the X chromosome. The discovery that a gene for color vision was located on the X chromosome was noted in 1911, but it took more than eighty years to find exactly where on the X chromosome this gene was located, and that there was more than one.

The Neitz Team

Then, barely eight years later, it became apparent that Dr. Nathans' team had discovered only a small number of genes for color vision. In 1995, on the 200th anniversary of John Dalton's publication of his explanation of inherited CVC, Jay Neitz, Ph.D., and Maureen Neitz, Ph.D., published their findings. The husband-and-wife team had made a startling discovery that seemed, for sure, to contradict the theory that had been held for 150 years. Along with their staff, they labored for ten years under the sponsorship of the National Institutes of Health and the departments of ophthalmology and cellular biology of the Medical College of Wisconsin, of the University of Wisconsin, at Milwaukee. They found that there are far more genes for color vision than previously thought, and that both colorblind and other persons have similar numbers of these genes. They also discovered that there are genes for far more color variations than previously thought, that color vision genes may vary in strength and placement on chromosomes, and that they may outshine other genes in their capacities. This discovery will doubtless lead to even wider research into color vision.

Clearly, at various times in the past 500 years, people—some quite well-known, and some who were rejected at first—have made efforts to untangle the mystery of human color vision. Not all of those who have made contributions to this study appear in this chapter. For all we know, somewhere someone has already noted what will be rediscovered in the future. The road to enlightenment has been long and confusing. Often it has been blocked by public misconceptions and refusal to be patient about finding proven facts. Little by little, more is being discovered. Slowly but surely, we are learning about the causes of faulty color vision. And, more and more, it has become increasingly apparent that colorblindness can be a serious side effect of various pollutants, diseases, and medications. Along with this increasing knowledge of color vision confusion come various tests that are now widely accepted, ways of understanding this handicap, and learning to live with it. All of these aspects of living with CVC are covered in the next section.

8

Color Vision Tests

Tests are tools. They are also very useful in diagnosing colorblindness. Unfortunately, quite a bit of negativity has been associated with taking any kind of test. So, with colorblindness tests, as with any test, remember that their main purpose is first to detect a physical condition—not a mental one—and then to take action from there. You cannot "fail" these tests, although you may discover that certain tasks or occupations are out of your reach.

There are many tests that have been developed over the years to detect colorblindness and color vision confusion. Some have been quite accurate, though time-consuming. Others have proven to be useless if given improperly, and others just have not stood the test of time. Due to the trials and errors of test-developers in the past we have learned a few important qualities that a test should have to succeed. The test should be:

- fast and easy to administer and interpret
- inexpensive and easy to transport
- valid and reliable in accord with daily life
- accurate in getting statistics as well as guiding the client

It should be made clear to the client before the test what is expected during the test, and what the intent of the test is in the first place. Also, the person administering the test should be properly trained, not only in giving the test but also in guiding the client after the results have been revealed. For instance, one should always consider that the very act of taking a test may be emotionally traumatic to some people, and discovering that they are color vision deficient may be just as traumatic. Their color vision confusion may be so mild, that they may have been unaware of it until that point. Proper diagnosis is therefore essential, and should be very carefully arrived at before making any conclusions. On the other hand, a client may be delighted to have found, at last, the reason for the ever-present visual confusion that has nothing to do with a poor mental state, a need for glasses, or an eye disease.

You may notice as you read through this chapter that most of the color vision tests were developed for, or by, the military institutions of one country or another. The military is known for its extremely thorough physical examinations, and color vision is a main concern during that exam. The reason for the military's strong interest in color vision testing is mainly safety. They have found that people with CVC may make excellent sharpshooters, while they would be dangerous pilots. Sharpshooters need to focus on one object or target, and "screen out" of their vision any other distractions. Colorblind people tend to have this ability naturally. Pilots, on the other hand, need to be able to distinguish colored lights on a control panel, in the air, and on the airport or other land panorama for landings with no tower guidance—a major problem for people with CVC. Through careful testing, the military is able to channel people to the positions to which they are best suited.

Keeping all of these points in mind, let's look at some of the tests that are available for detecting color vision confusion.

NAGEL ANOMALOSCOPE TEST

This test was developed by a German scientist by the name of W.A. Nagel in 1907. It is a very exacting test, and gives very exacting results. It is the only test that can distinguish all four types of CVC. It was the first test to offer information about blue color vision confusion. (Blue color vision confusion was later shown to be a potential indicator of the state of health of the person tested.) The Nagel Anomaloscope Test also can detect complete lack of color vision.

One of this test's major drawbacks is that it is rather confusing to explain to the average person, and takes a long time to administer correctly—under very precise conditions and lighting—for this reason, it is used mainly for research purposes, rather than for everyday diagnosis.

FARNSWORTH-MUNSELL 100 HUE TEST

This test was designed by Dean Farnsworth of the Department of Psychology at New York University in 1943. It mainly tests for the colors blue, violet, and green. Its name comes from the fact that it tests for 100 hues. The streamlined series actually has only 85 samples. It can be obtained from the Graphic Arts Technical Foundation in Pittsburgh, PA, which serves the graphic arts community, but sells the product to others as well. It is a somewhat tedious test and requires special lighting. It was designed as a test for research-type laboratory situations.

To explain how a test of this kind is arrived at, Farnsworth stated that any screening test of color vision is a kind of "trick" as he called it. He said that the test takes advantage of some weaknesses that those who have inherited color vision confusion are known to have in seeing colors. He said that in order to help those who have color vision confusion one must be able to determine just where the confusion lies, and for this testing, must take place with some tools. This test was such a tool.

FALANT (FARNSWORTH-LANTERN) EYE TEST

This test, which was at one point called the New London Navy Lantern Test, is the "definitive" test used by the United States Navy, Coast Guard, and Air Force. It is the test one must be able to complete properly in order to get a ship captain's license or an airplane pilot's license. The FALANT test became the official test used by the United States Navy in 1945.

The FALANT test replicates, in clinical conditions, the task of identifying and distinguishing red, green, and white lights in the distance. In other words, the test is intended to substitute for what might be seen in the distance while on a ship or airplane, but the test is administered indoors under specific lighting conditions. The colors that were selected for testing are those one would have to be able to decipher as buoys at sea, lights on ships, and lights on planes. On ships, one color is used for the port side of the boat and another for the starboard side, to indicate left and right. On airplanes you see these colors on the tips of wings. (On planes it indicates right or left to assure close encounters do not take place in the air.)

During this test, light beams are projected onto a screen in pairs. The

THE COST OF BLUNDERS

You may have noticed by now the strong emphasis placed on properly administering these tests. You may wonder what difference it makes if someone is tested and diagnosed as being colorblind when he or she is not, or the other way around—being told one has perfect color vision when actually the person has CVC. The United States Air Force now knows the repercussions of improper testing. In 1987 the United States Air Force was sued by a student from the Memphis State University Air Force R.O.T.C. program.

The Memphis State College student had joined the Air Force Reserve Officers Training Corps program on the college campus after taking a complete physical, including a color vision test. He was aiming to become a pilot. This student, Andrew Jackson Woodrick, even landed in military jail due to this mix-up. When his case went to court it became a news article that appeared on the front page of the New York Times.

Mr. Woodrick had enlisted after taking a test while he was a sophomore at Memphis State University. The physical was given by arrangement with the Air Force R.O.T.C. unit to determine if he was qualified to become a pilot candidate.

He was deemed fit, and he began his R.O.T.C. studies in September of 1981. He attended classes diligently and passed written exams. In October of 1982, he took a precommission physical to verify his suitability for pilot training. This time, the color vision test indicated that he was colorblind. He was told by his superiors that as a result, he was no longer eligible for pilot's training.

But Woodrick insisted that he had contracted with the R.O.T.C. to become a pilot, and that in effect, he had contracted to take on missions the military would choose once he became a pilot. He fully intended to abide by that contract, and insisted that the Air Force R.O.T.C. abide by it as well.

After he was told that he was not fit to become a pilot, he did not attend the R.O.T.C. preparatory classes. But he was told to continue to attend these classes. He would not, nor did he cash in the stipend that the R.O.T.C. offers students.

For not attending classes, he was threatened with court martial. He tried to explain to the commanding officer why he had stopped attending classes, and had expected to be decommissioned and to be dropped from the program. But this is not what happened.

> He certainly could have used the money the stipend offered. But because he wouldn't, he had to take fewer classes per semester so that he could work long hours to pay for his college education. Another vision test was ordered by the Air Force, and he failed to appear. He was told to report to active duty as an enlisted man after he returned from his Christmas break during his senior year in 1982. He refused, and as a result he was locked up in a windowless room in the Lakeland Air Force Base in San Antonio Texas, facing a court martial.
>
> He decided to sue the Air Force for breach of contract and harassment. Woodrick lost his senior year of college, and graduation. He was the son of a World War II bomber navigator. He had wanted to serve his country as a pilot, but he was being handled as a criminal.
>
> The case dragged on for six years, and court costs mounted on both sides. All of this could have been avoided if the original color vision test had been properly administered and clearly explained.

pair might be red and green, red and red, red and white, green and green, green and white, or white and white. The FALANT test was developed with funding from the United States Navy as a substitute for the Edridge-Green Lantern Test that was used by the British Navy. Due to the outbreak of the Second World War, the British test became unavailable in the United States and another one had to be substituted.

As with all of these CVC tests, proper testing with the FALANT test is crucial. In the period between 1981 and 1991, an unusually high number of poorly administered tests were recorded. These tests were done by people who had no grasp of just how delicate a problem color vision confusion could be in the high-tech military world. The test was not administered by military medical personnel, but rather, under contract from the reserve and R.O.T.C. (Reserve Officers Training Corps) by local optometrists and other "qualified" personnel.

This shoddy attention to the FALANT testing method was a result of the military cost-cutting efforts—it was rationalized that local testing would be far more convenient to the person who was to be tested. Otherwise, in many cases, those who were to be tested would have to travel long distances for the test, and this could prove to be a financial burden.

Like the Nagel Test, the FALANT test is rarely administered to the general public.

ISHIHARA TEST

As we noted, most of the tests for color vision began in military settings or were funded by the military of one country or another. The Ishihara Test was developed at the Imperial Military Academy of Tokyo, Japan, by an instructor named Shinobu Ishihara.

The Ishihara Test is the "granddaddy" of all color vision tests used today, although admittedly Ishihara's test plates were based on the plates produced by Stilling more than 100 years ago, and Stilling was an American. It is distributed by the Kanehera Publishing Company, a medical reference books publisher in Tokyo, Japan.

The Ishihara Test was once a long, drawn out process that often tired the eyes of the tested person as well as the tester, which wasn't good for the results of the test. People would have to match one hundred squares of colors of various gradation of values up to the most pastel-whitish, then go on to match another batch with other colors, and then start the whole process again with another set of cards, until all types of combinations were checked. But from the time it was first introduced in the U.S. in 1924 to this day, this test has been hailed as the most exact, most delicate, and most accurate in detecting even mild cases, pinpointing moderate cases, and verifying serious cases.

Today it is a test that can be administered in regular adequate daylight, with no special lamps, and is made up of eight test plates. Where once the pseudoisochromatic plate was a reworked copy of the Ishihara test, today the Ishihara test has been tailored to be short like the modern Pseudoisochromatic Test. Today, even the Japanese do not have the luxury of the amount of time they once had to devote to the test (which would be taken almost at the pace of a Japanese tea ceremony). But the colors of the Ishihara test plates seem more vibrant than those of the pseudoisochromatic test. Because the designs in this test are composed of small "blobs," this is sometimes called "the dot test."

If the Ishihara Test or the Pseudoisochromatic Test is given for screening a person's potential employment and this person "fails," an opportunity should be given to retake the test to establish the degree of color vision confusion he or she has before excluding this person from the job. This is because not all jobs really need full color vision, and people with mild cases of inherited CVC may be well qualified for the job in question.

AO/H.R.R. PSEUDOISOCHROMATIC TEST

This is the test that is used most often. It was developed along the lines of the Ishihara Test. So why was it developed? Perhaps because Japan was at war with America during the Second World War, making the Ishihara test plates unavailable. The AO/H.R.R. Pseudoisochromatic Test was originally developed with funding from the United States military in 1943, and was not actually available to the public until ten years later—almost as if it were a military secret.

The "AO" in the name of this test stands for the American Optical Company that once handled the distribution of the test. (It is now handled by a number of companies including the Richmond Products Company of Boca Raton, Florida, a company that is a distributor of all sorts of optical supplies).

The "H.R.R." stands for Hardy, Rand, and Ritter, the three researchers who developed this as a practical test for general use. "Pseudo-iso-chromatic" means apparently or falsely equal colors. In other words, the colors are chosen to fall within the design or diagram in such a way that those who might have trouble seeing them will be trapped. They appear to be equal to someone who would not see their color, for they are equal in chroma of color, and intensity of the colors. "Pseudo" means "false or substitute," "iso" means "same," and chromatic stands for what it sounds like. Put them all together and you get "substitute-same-chroma."

If you had full color vision and looked at a sample plate from this test, you would see a number, composed of blobs of one color, appear clearly somewhere in the center of a circle of blobs of another color. The first plate shown at the beginning of the test can be seen clearly by those who are colorblind as well as others, because it is made up of the two colors that even those who have inherited color vision confusion, and do not have total blindness to colors, can see. The colors are orange (which is sometimes referred to as amber these days) and a grey-blue. Only two colors or hues are found in each of the following test plates. But the numbers or designs you have to find are different, and the colors of the background and the design to be found may vary from plate to plate. This is done to find out which colors look the same to you. This also tests at which intensity of chroma your vision might become confused. Because the Ishihara and this test look so similar, this test is also sometimes called "the dot test."

The test is to be given in a specific sequence and under specific lighting conditions. The test plates are not meant simply as something anyone should toy with. It would be sad if the test were given incorrectly by someone who is not experienced, because a false diagnosis can be devastating.

Even in 1945, the authors of the Pseudoisochromatic Test, Hardy, Rand, and Ritter, asked that serious attention be given to how the test is administered. They found that, at times, there was critical disregard for lighting in the environment where the test was given. Worse yet, the test givers were often incompetent and careless. Their interpretation of the results and misapplication of the information were harmful and wasteful.

TITMUS II VISION TESTER COLOR PERCEPTION TEST

The TITMUS II Vision Tester Color Perception Test is a relatively new test that is produced by computer with fiber optics. It uses photographically reproduced pseudoisochromatic designs, and can test one eye at a time. The person tested looks into a stereoscopic unit. The chin rests on a base, and the image comes on only when the forehead touches a pad on the top of the unit.

Such units can often be found in doctor's offices. They are also lightweight enough to be moved from one location to another, as they weigh only about 12 pounds, and they can be plugged in anywhere a computer outlet can be found. There are two settings to choose from, for nearsighted people as well as for people with regular vision.

This instrument is easy to use and practical in design. It can be used anytime. Testers do not have to be highly trained. Among the drawbacks is the fact that anyone with less than 20/70 vision in both eyes may fail the test—not because of an inability to see what is on the plates due to color vision problems, but because of regular vision problems.

There is a series of plates, or you can use just one test plate. The one test plate most often available at doctor's offices is one that has six samples on it. Six different designs or numbers in them are to be deciphered. They are on a black background, but they are framed in a yellow border that vies for attention, even in the vision of someone who has regular color vision—another definite drawback.

It is a quick test, and it is better than nothing. It is attractive because it appears to be high-tech, but its value is limited because it only tests for red/green deficiencies and it is not highly accurate.

STILL IN THE WORKS

There are many tests still being developed that may one day help us study different aspects of color vision confusion. There is a new test that is aimed at detecting the effects of aging on color vision. It is meant for research on planning safer and more functional environments for elderly people. Meanwhile, researchers are making advances with tests in various other areas that are affected by color-blindness. The following are still being developed:

- The Mandola Colorvision Screening Test for preschool- and kinder-garten-age children is among the tests being developed for screening young children.
- Tests are being developed for measuring light sensitivity in relation to chroma in color vision.
- A table-top device for measuring tritanopia, or blue-yellow sensitivity produced by Spec Rx, Inc., under license from Georgia Tech, is being developed to determine just how well this color vision abnormality can be used as a guide to diagnosis of illnesses. This is particularly useful for quickly testing groups for diabetes.
- A test is being developed by a fiber optics specialist who is color-blind. It may help those who have inherited color vision confusion gauge to just what degree they are "different" from those who have regular color vision, and to measure their cases against others. A better understanding of this condition—a life-long visual distur-bance—could develop.

COLOR-BIASED TESTING

It should be noted that some psychological tests that include colors have, until recently, not taken into account colorblindness or testing for color vision confusion before administering the test. This is true of the Rorschach Test, which is used for determining emotional and intellectual personality traits, and is now given in colors.

Also, the Irlen Method of dealing with dyslexia, by way of having a person read through a transparent sheet of color-tinted plastic, has not included a color vision test before considering the prescription of the tinted sheet.

The Luscher Test, touted as a "deep" personality test by its devel-oper, Dr. Max Luscher of Switzerland, was introduced into the United

States in 1971, and given a big spread in *Life* magazine.

It is a test in which people have to place eight colored cards in the order they think best answers some personality question, and then they can check to find out what it means in a book. This book contains the following claim about people who are colorblind:

Color blindness makes no difference. The instinctive response to color in terms of contrast makes the Luscher Test valid even in cases of defective color vision or even actual color blindness, since the acceptability of some color is somatically (from Greek *soma*, body; somatic therefore means *having to do with the body*) related to the degree to which anabolism and catabolism is needed by an organism.

But the use of colors in the test is very biased. Still, the book went on to state that tests were made by L. Steinke to prove that this test is valid even for people who are colorblind. This is very hard to believe and such claims have not been available for verification. The test is, however, still used at times.

In 1988, two Canadian researchers, Stanley Coren and Ralph Hakstian introduced a very different test. Instead of showing color plates or lights to the person taking the test, the person actually answers a series of questions in his or her own home. The questionnaire asks questions about life situations that colorblind people might normally have difficulty with. Depending on the score of the test, the instructions on the test might then suggest that the person have a more extensive test done to determine the degree of color vision confusion.

This test makes a lot of sense because it assumes that people who have experienced color vision confusion have an idea that something about their vision is "off." Giving them a test like the Ishihara Test may be useful, but it may be all the more useful for people to screen themselves, in the comfort of their own homes, before they face the challenge of being rejected for whatever task or job.

A FINAL COMMENT ON TESTS

As you can see, tests for colorblindness are very necessary. It is important to detect color vision deficiencies early, both to avoid dangerous situations as well as to avoid individual embarrassment and grief. Testing earlier may also help researchers better understand how colorblindness affects different aspects of life—such as school grades or job performance—and possibly make adjustments for those situations, so that those particular environments are no longer biased towards those with full color vision. You can request a color vision test during your next routine eye exam. If your doctor can't do it, he or she should be able to refer you to someone who can. As long as the technology exists to detect color vision confusion, we should make the most of it.

9

Learning, Memory, & Color Vision

You may ask how learning and memory have anything to do with color vision confusion. Well, it's really the other way around—color vision affects how we learn and remember things. Learning depends on association of information. New information is absorbed and mentally digested until it becomes useful to the mind. This information is then added to details previously saved in the memory. Color is an integral part of this information.

Looking at unfamiliar objects is one of the most trying of all visual situations, but it occurs far more frequently than we assume. You look at unfamiliar objects when you go shopping, visit a museum or festival, find your way when traveling, try to repair an appliance, or go to a party. The unfamiliar makes the eyes and mind work overtime. It causes mental fatigue, especially if you have to guess about things that your eye and mind cannot register, such as colors.

No matter how hard a person with CVC looks at an object, and no matter what substitute color the person's mind registers, the person does not get the same information that others get with just one glance. For instance, the color of a person's skin can help you determine if someone has a fever, is embarrassed, has a sunburn, or is feeling ill. The color of the sky may tell you what the weather has in store. The intensity or degree of a color can help you tell how far away an object is—you can place it in relation to other objects of other colors. By looking at a traffic light, you can tell if you should stop, go, or slow down. Color sight enhances visual experiences and aids in our comprehension and thus our response.

HOW DO WE REMEMBER THINGS?

Memory is collected information, including visual and other sensory details. Visual memory is registered in the mind by what Jeremy Campbell calls "visual noise." In his book *The Grammatical Man*, Campbell points out that visual noise is anything that causes a visual distraction, and stimulates the mind to focus strongly on a stimulus, thus recording it in its mental file. The visual noise to which we are most attracted varies from individual to individual, depending on such things as our interests and previous experiences. But visual noise is the catalyst that, in the end, determines the visual experiences you remember. Obviously, colors are an important source of visual noise. Consider, for instance, that if you had never tasted chocolate, a brown square in a box would mean nothing to you. Furthermore, memories may be stored in a confused manner or may be inaccurately retrieved if needed pre-information (color) is missing or if the mental image is confused.

It has been determined that visual perception, and our understanding of what we see and experience, as well as our decision-making, is based on "betting on probabilities." But in order to determine the probabilities, we have to use our memories, our *recall*. This recall is a storage area in our brains that has stored information and experiences. Our recall aids us in everyday situations to avoid accidents, to make choices, to remember names, and for many more things that we take for granted. For example, when we see pizza, we might remember what pizza tastes like, but more importantly, we assume "hot!". Someone who had never seen a pizza would not recognize the possibility of being burned by one, because it isn't in their *recall*. A good example of this recall would be choosing jellybeans. Most of us know that orange jellybeans are orange-flavored, yellow ones are lemon-flavored, green ones are lime-flavored, black ones are licorice-flavored, and so on. If you have trouble processing these colors in your brain, you might have difficulty remembering which flavors you liked, or you might avoid an otherwise good flavor because the color looked unappetizing to you. If we do not recall colors, we miss a significant amount of information, and therefore we are more unsure in our "predictions" of what we're really seeing and how to react to it.

In order to remember information, it is best if there is an organized package of information, or information in some systematic form. It is far harder to remember random bits of information. The brain likes knowing what a thing is, how it looks, and what it's used for. It likes to file information in units of some form. The more detailed information that is available in one's memory, the more ability the mind has to pull out appropriate aspects of memory when needed.

The mind can also choose what details to forget. If you remember how a tree looks by using texture, size, and shape, you may be able to forget color. If you are colorblind, you may have no other choice. Someone who has not managed to store the detailed information that colors offer may have to think longer, guess more, and be prepared for errors. For instance, think of how a smart person with CVC would react to a color monitor on a computer. It would take that person extra time and thought to process information on the screen that people with full color vision take for granted. What if the person with CVC can't see the information on the screen at all? Pressing one key when a screen that looks blank is actually on can cause tremendous problems. Just think of the consequences of errors—punishment, shame, loss of self confidence, not to mention wasted time. This can be very discouraging for anyone.

Smart people find ways to circumvent the mental short circuit caused by CVC. Others may tune out or choose other activities that they can deal with. For this reason, you may find that people who have colorblindness may avoid playing certain board games or doing certain jobs. They may react a bit more slowly in doing some tasks. No one wants to make errors. Mistakes can be both tiring and frustrating.

Basically, the mechanism of visual memory is universal. We all tend to record things in our minds in similar ways unless, that is, there has been some dramatic disruption requiring a different process. Activities that require our visual memories—be it writing, drawing, or telling descriptive tales—usually reflect what is in our minds, what we use as our personal encyclopedia.

Now take a minute and try this: Take a piece of paper and a pencil and draw a duck. Never mind how it looks. No one except you will see your duck. If you prefer, you can draw the duck on this page with your finger, without leaving a trace for anyone to see. Go ahead, don't be shy. You do remember what a duck looks like, right? Most people do. Whether they have seen a real duck or not, people visualize a certain animal in their minds when they hear the word that means "duck" in the language they speak. You already see your duck, don't you? It already exists in your mind's eye.

I have not seen your duck, but, in all probability, it is standing sideways. It is facing left if you are right-handed and right if you are left-handed. If you sketched it, you started at the head, and the line continued down the neck to the back tail feathers. Right?

Am I guessing? No. I have tried this experiment on people of all walks of life; all nationalities, religions, and cultural backgrounds; all educational and economic levels. They all react similarly. To project what is probable, one has to have information that is based on recurrence. My experience has shown that people's tendency to face objects in a given direction is fairly constant. In fact, the pictographs of the ancient Egyptians faced sideways as did the drawings the cavemen left us.

Let's take the experiment one step further. If I ask you to draw a duck and a pond, chances are you will make a circle and in the middle there will be a duck without feet. We all assume that the duck actually has feet, but they are not seen because they are in the water.

Back to our ducks. If you were asked to place a fence in front of the pond, this might cause some discomfort because it might obliterate part of your duck. Why was it acceptable for the duck's legs not to show in the pond, but not acceptable for the duck to be partly out of view? The reason is simple. We need to have as much visual information as we can get, and are uncomfortable when we lose too much. Of course, some people will need to pictorially acknowledge the existence of the feet, making the duck appear to walk on water. some people objected to the showing of less than whole persons in the early days of television and home videos. To them, talking heads were unacceptable.

Through experience, we have all discovered that communication is possible even without all the visual information. A side view gives us at least half the information. However, when it comes to the legs, chances are you will show that the duck has two, not one, not four.

We need reference. We need to have information in units. We can then subtract whatever details we wish from the unit, but the unit must at least be in our minds. Storing information in your mind is not always intended or conscious. Most often, we do not consider whether or not we should commit something to memory. In fact, there are some things that are not so vivid in our memories. But memory and the ability to recall are the basis for acquiring knowledge that can be used in the future. Our minds combine what is happening now with information stored in our memory bank to let us know what will probably happen next and what to do immediately.

Association of words, feelings, details, and amounts is important. The clustering of units of information is important. If we lack some of this information we get the response that psychologists have labeled TOT (tip of tongue) memory. In such a situation, and I am sure you have experienced this, you can recall the incident, person, or item as well as the location, and the meaning, but you are missing the specifics—the name of the person or item or place. In some cases, you remember just about everything but cannot recall whether it was blue or . . . .

Colors are one of the very dominant cues that the mind uses as a bit of unit information to remember things. Visual information usually contains data on location, color, and row (or relationship to the rest of the information). If you do not have color information, or if it is garbled, you miss retrieval cues for complete recall of information.

When we have only disjointed memory or when our memory has information that is not unified, we are considered absent-minded. It is not that our minds are absent, but that coherent memory recall is not total, or is so weak that it is ignored by the mind as useless.

For people who are colorblind, all visual information is a bit garbled. They are uncertain of one visual clue that others take for granted. This is one reason that many people do not like to play board games, or video games, especially games like Trivial Pursuit that have color-coded material. For this reason, some will be seen as hyperactive: at least when they are in action they need not consider long forgotten details of the past. For this reason, some students cannot concentrate on the printed page, they do not see the material as clear, memorable, and useful.

Consider Vinnie Testaverde. In the 1980s he was a star quarterback for the Tampa Bay Buccaneers in the National Football League (NFL), who seemed to be having memory lapses. He was hailed as one of the most promising "properties," and his future appeared very bright. But, for some reason, he kept throwing his fantastic passes into the arms of the "enemy." He was puzzled, and so were those who saw what he did.

I bet you can guess the reason for his problems by now. Everybody on the field looked pretty much the same to him. He could not tell the uniforms apart—not because he was hasty, not because he was stupid, not because he ignored the game plan, but because he is colorblind.

Who thinks about football in relation to colorblindness? Hardly anyone. But once the cause was understood, a solution was found.

The solution was to have one team wear dark colored pants and light shirts, while the other team wears the reverse combination. Or else, have one team wear one color uniform with the player's number in a contrasting color, and have the other team wear a very different color that is of very different color value contrast, not only color hue cotrast.

We know that Vinnie Testaverde did not forget what to do. He was not absent-minded. He was not sloppy. He was confused as to how to distinguish between similarly dressed people who were running around on the field. He was missing a big visual cue—color.

COLORS AS REFERENCE WORDS AND TRIGGERS FOR RECALL

Advertisers spend a lot of money researching and utilizing the colors and symbols that adults and young children will be attracted to so that Mommy will have to buy a given item. Who, in all the world, cannot tell you the colors of the McDonald's arches and what they indicate? Well, they could tell you what the design of the McDonald's arches indicate even from afar, but not all could tell you the colors, although they may have learned by now, from hearing about it, that they are the "golden" arches.

Adults usually know how to read, but when you grab a container of milk, and you know that the one with the purple-colored print is the low-fat milk, you need not even take time to read. You just head for the milk section of the supermarket and reach for the container. If, that is, you can tell purple from blue. These colors that are used as easy recognition for products are "triggers." But when different manufacturers use different color triggers for the same product, triggers can backfire and frustrate the consumers.

Even those who have full color vision will agree that the mind does not like the fact that one company has low-fat milk in blue containers, and another has the same item in green or purple. It annoys people who see all colors. Imagine how confusing it is for those who confuse colors! It can be mind boggling!

The mind does not like randomness, it likes order and consistency. We like to hear the same traditional hymns when going to church or synagogue. That is what we expected to hear and, that's what soothes us and gives us a sense of security in constancy. We look for the traffic light to turn from green, to yellow, to red, and know which will turn next. For someone who is colorblind this is of great significance. Once the sequence is learned, it can be guessed at if not seen totally, and you gear yourself to cross the street. But if the sequence is changed, you are stumped, because there are no reliable color cues available to you.

Not a day goes by without the need to refer to colors. We use colors to code books and reference materials that contain information that we need to retrieve. We recognize the subway stop, the bus we take to work, our cars, and our bicycles by their colors. We choose food—a sizzling steak, a tossed salad, a cake, a drink—by the appeal of their colors. We choose our wardrobe based in large part on colors. By looking at a fruit and the color of its skin, we can usually tell if the fruit is ripe, hard or soft, or if it will be sweet or tart. Knowing such information before we bite into the fruit and have to deal with a mouthful can be very helpful. Like it or not, we also are attracted to other people on the basis of eye color, hair color, and complexion color as much as by other details.

Parents and teachers often are unaware of the significance of color and of the problems that result from confusion of "expected" visual information.

Everyday Triggers

Names for colors are a part of all languages. From ruby red to black as pitch, color terminology does more than tell us how pretty an object is. Colors can be used to describe feelings such as love, hate, warmth, sadness, and so forth. And when we see red and green ribbons or orange and black decorations, or when we receive red and white hearts, we can instantly identify the holiday as well as the spirit. Colors are an important part of humanity's unspoken form of communication. Colors provide information, a frame of reference, and a trigger for recall. So, when distortions exist, confused messages reach the brain. And, because the messages are confused, they are either not stored in the memory, or they are stored with jumbled details that will prove confusing if recalled.

Does Christmas remind you of the color orange? Could the star of David be violet? Could Navy uniforms be brown? Perhaps they could. But the colors we associate with them were selected for good reason. They are psychological triggers.

People who are colorblind often learn that the images stored in their memories are jumbled, and they have to take time to guess on correct "probabilities." Is a small round object an olive or a maraschino cherry? If it is on a buffet platter, it probably is a food and it probably tastes good to someone. But will it taste as expected? If you're not sure what it is, perhaps you'd better pass. Colorblind people often do pass or opt out of various situations.

Sometimes individuals will hesitate to ask questions, especially when their confusion is connected with a color they cannot decipher. They fear having to explain that. They do not want to ask questions that may appear "stupid," but they do not want to explain why they cannot see some of the cues and colors.

Just imagine the mistakes, confusion, and wasted effort experienced by those who cannot see the colors others take for granted. The blue stuff in the bottle is window wash, the green stuff is antifreeze, the red stuff is ketchup, and so on. We learn to differentiate these cues and memorize them for the next time we will need to use these items. In everyday situations, it is safer and easier for someone with CVC to take a few extra seconds to read a label, if there is one available. These cues help to make us independent individuals. Recognizing the cues is what a child strives for on the way to adulthood. The process of learning the cues begins in infancy.

THE AGES OF MEMORY

Color affects each individual at every stage of life. The ability to see color may determine whether or not a baby responds to certain stimuli, the way a child learns to read, or the career choice a young adult makes. It may also affect an older person's relationship with his or her spouse of many years, and his or her ability to be independent and healthy.

Infancy

The effort to learn to differentiate and to memorize begins not in kindergarten, but in the crib. True, no one expects much from a baby in a crib, but the child learns to differentiate images, to recognize parents or other familiar faces, to recognize pets, toys, and bottles. Until recently, few of us were aware of just how much goes on in an infant's head. Much transpires in the development of the infant's eyes and in the development of the connections between sight and memory. All of this affects learning.

How many colored objects have you seen hanging above a crib or carriage to entertain the infant from birth on? From the beginning, parents push color recognition. They know that children have been left back in kindergarten for not knowing their colors. There is, however, no proof that infants see colors distinctly at the crib stage. We know that it takes some time before infants actually see anything clearly. Color vision may or may not develop at the same rate. It has been estimated that some colors register with infants far better others.

Experiments conducted to determine which colors four-month-old infants are most attracted to surprised those who had expected a wide range of interest. The infants tended to choose a limited range. Pure red and blue were given much more time and attention than other colors. When the experiment was repeated, with one other color along side, the infants seemed to be attracted to green and yellow as well, but only if the colors were pure in their intensity, with strong chroma, and not mixed, as a blue-green might be, or a violet-red might be.

Little research has been done on what colors infants see. It is really hard to judge. Certainly, they cannot speak and tell us what colors they see. Motion may be far more interesting to them.

In Kindergarten

By the time a child is in kindergarten, the learning process speeds up. Colors become adjectives, tools of specific verbal communication regarding selecting food, asking for a toy, or using a crayon. By then, children are expected to learn to differentiate colors, to know their names, and to associate these colors with other objects in their lives. The use of colors predominates the learning environment.

Holidays have associated decorations of specific colors; Christmas is not orange and black. Or is it? If you are red-green colorblind, red becomes black and green can be orange. Imagine the reaction to a child whose Christmas cards are black and orange! And what about the tried and true red, white, and blue that we connect with the flag, what is that to a colorblind child? It can be black, violet, and green.

The child's cubby or locker, in which personal things are stored, is often color-coded so that it can be found by the child who cannot yet read his or her name. What happens if the cubby is moved?

It is rare to give a child a book illustrated in a very limited number of colors. Crayons, paper, and peg boards come in an array of the colors that a child may not be able to identify or ask for. What happens if you have been told that green is "go" and red is "stop" but you do not see these colors? Often children are considered inattentive, or too lazy to memorize information, and sometimes they may be considered downright stupid if they make the same mistake over and over again. Color vision confusion can cause turmoil at the very time that the child needs to be focused on learning. Many men have told me that their first moment of feeling worthless because of colorblindness was in kindergarten.

Colors can be a means of expressing feelings or preferences. Often, when a child exhibits odd choices of color use, a kindergarten teacher will assume that the child is creative. But the misinterpretation of colorblindness is usually not so positive. A constant attraction to black is often translated by adults to mean the child may be mentally or emotionally disturbed. Rarely will a teacher assume that this child actually sees colors in a different way. Rarely do educators or parents understand that the child would delight in seeing colors like the rest of the kids do. The colorblind child does not like having to deal with odd questions and having to explain himself all the time, or to be unable to play some video game as well as others because he cannot follow the colored images.

Primary Grades

By first grade, if a child does not know the colors, it is assumed that the child is slow. Very few teachers have been trained to consider the matter of color vision confusion, to recognize the need for testing or to administer tests. At this age, the child who has color vision confusion begins to get odd responses from others, sometimes giggles, and even jeers. By the second grade, a child's unusual use of color is less likely to be considered a flight of fancy and more likely to be considered willful or nonconforming.

In first grade, it is time for learning to read. Color codes are used as cues when written language is introduced. One of the aspects of quick reading is fluency in naming. Naming is the ability to translate the visual image of an object into its verbal label, and early reading skill depends on the speed or fluency with which this translation takes place. Educational researchers have revealed in a number of experiments that 70 percent of slow readers were halted by misconnections where colors were involved.

Although the statistics seem to improve with the age of the child, the fact is that those who still showed poor naming capacity when related to color or colored objects, were not, as one might suspect, tested for color vision. At least, no such action was reported.

Many of the books one can find on the library shelves in regard to the problems of learning among young children point to hyperactivity and the inability to concentrate. There is now material about dyslexia, but rarely does one find information that suggests that if a child's concentration wanders, perhaps this child does not see the colors that are pointed out.

No suggestions are made to test hyperactive children for color vision. If anything, there are suggestions that adding colors to the material hyperactive children use will help keep their attention on the material. But there is no proof of that. Nor are there any statistics about color vision confusion in hyperactive children because there has been no wide-scale testing. Perhaps there should be. Consider the stories you've heard of deaf students who are not tested when they do not respond properly; they are simply shouted at. "Shouting" colors to someone who does not see them and cannot readily explain what he does not see is like shouting at the deaf. We have learned, in recent years, that such behavior is fruitless. Yet we blast colors everywhere.

Today, the term "learning disability" generally refers to disability of grasping the concepts of reading and mathematics. Dyslexia is given a great deal of attention because the condition affects how a person sees words, thus, reading and math abilities are affected. In dyslexia, people confuse the location of letters and numbers and sometimes see them backwards or swimming around. You cannot do math on paper very well under such conditions. It is not lack of intellectual ability to grasp the words or the mathematical concepts that hampers dyslexics, it is only their inability to see or write the material.

Yet, cognition and memory recall is the basis of learning and use of what has been learned. Even intelligence tests contain a section on color recognition. And, if we cannot see the colors properly, or we have to answer in a particular colored box and we do not know where it is, we appear dumb for not knowing and not answering the question. All too often, the quick fix is the prescription of medication or psychological counseling for someone who does not "live up to expectations." Neither of these solutions will make a person who has a color vision problem see colors better, nor will the child be able to respond in situations where color vision is needed to aid in decision making.

Sometimes, it may seem as if the most important decision a child needs to make is what color gumball he or she wants, but it is crucial that young children learn certain colors to avoid dangerous situations. For instance, learning to "cross on the green," learning that red appliances are often very hot and dangerous, or perhaps learning a specific color code at school can mean the difference between getting in trouble or even life and death.

If "mistakes" are made often enough in the young years, and if a child is chastised for making these mistakes, the inner pain begins. The name calling starts. The self's protective inner-shield begins to grow. Fearful of name calling and embarrassments, a child may become very shy or act out. A child may recoil, hesitating to ask questions for which he doesn't get clear answers, or the child may become so bossy that no one will dare to argue with him. A colorblind child may also tune out of the process of learning. The child may become a "clown," enticing laughter so that he, at last, knows why others are laughing at him. Adults may then assume that the child is looking for attention and that he is a trouble maker. Such a child will lose time doing his tasks and disturb others, keeping them from accomplishing theirs. This may be part of the strategy. Such a child may well think, "If others do not manage to do things, then I will not be that different. I won't be an outcast." In fact, this may not be too far from the truth, but, ultimately, the reaction of others—annoyance and disengagement from other children—reinforces negative self-image and improper behavior.

There have been some studies on the relationship of colorblindness and personality types, but they have shown that there is no great personality deviation among those who are colorblind in contrast to those who are not. However, it would be useful to have statistics on the numbers of young people who have landed in the criminal justice system not because of personality defects, but, at least in part, because of color vision confusion. These young people may have been designated as, or seen themselves as, failures because of their problem.

Furthermore, they may have missed absorbing basic knowledge upon which further school studies rest, and been classified as slow or disruptive in their early years in school.

The Teen Years

In the teen years, young people are still developing a strong sense of self-confidence and a feeling for "who they are." These years are known for "learning the hard way." But imagine how much harder it can be for a colorblind teen. This is a time when young people can establish a sense of independence and responsibility. This is also a time when teens feel a strong need to express themselves and exert their individuality. One might develop an artistic side; get a job, possibly even start a small business; start dressing to follow their own likes and dislikes; girls might start wearing make-up, and maybe even dying their hair. In any of these situations, CVC can become quite apparent, and, if it is not recognized as color vision confusion, the young adult may be classified as a special education student, which can stigmatize a child and have a tremendous impact on the child's behavior. All of these choices are based on what has been learned so far, and stored in memory.

Self-esteem is an important consideration in these years. A young person who loses a job because of a color-coding mix-up may give up on authority figures, or worse—give up on himself. A young person who chooses an outlandish color for hair or clothing can instantly become a social outcast among peers. His or her artwork may be in colors that are seen as depressing or odd, which can cause a young adult to be stereotyped as somehow mentally disturbed.

Any of the above scenarios can cause a developing teen to become delinquent, or perhaps an introvert, either way setting the person up for possible failure. If the person is tested for CVC, and discovers the problem early enough, he or she can learn coping skills for such situations. The teen can learn that others who are "normal" also have it.

Criticism might not necessarily come from peers either, often it comes from parents who do not understand their child's special needs. I know of a case where a father considered his sixteen-year-old son a sissy because he didn't want to drive at night. It was bad enough that in early childhood the boy was afraid of the dark, but in teen years? And when he had an accident at night, was he drinking, or perhaps worse? He claims he wasn't, he just did not see the other driver's blinker, or the traffic light. It was assumed that the boy was just an irresponsible driver. His claim was never checked out.

This same boy's father, an avid sportsman, was also annoyed that his son would not join him in target practice. The son said he could not see the red target, to which the father replied that if the boy paid attention, he would do just fine.

The father's disappointment grew into anger. He could not comprehend what the boy was telling him. He didn't understand how the boy couldn't see things properly if he didn't need glasses.

As if his father's anger wasn't enough for this young person to bear, his parents soon got a divorce. His mother had tired of being blamed by his father for causing her son's "birth defects." This caused a secret guilt in the son, for feeling that he was the cause of the divorce. This affected the boy to the extent that he feared making errors and therefore chose to refrain from doing things he was not very sure of. He eventually found a place for himself in the workforce as a systems analyst. No colors are needed in this occupation, and you can test if you are right, because the machine will tell you without making nasty remarks, snickering at you, or rejecting you if you are not on the mark.

Fortunately, this story has a happy ending. As it turned out, the boy eventually fell in love with a girl who understood, in spite of the fact that he told her that he loved her "green" complexion—he intended to say pink, of course, but his mind had registered the color as the same, without any memory notation that green is not a color one would want one's skin to be. He confided to me that he was impressed that she did not use that colored cream that is sometimes used to hide pimples or other blemishes on the face by teenagers. (Since he is clearly attuned to variations of tones, the cream blotches that have been smeared on in various places on the face seem worse to him than real blotches that he often cannot see at all. (The cream blotches give girls a clown look as his eyes see them.)

As Adults

Some only discover that they are colorblind late in their lives. Oh, they may have known their vision was different, but they did not let on. These people may have hidden in "safe" jobs where they could make a good living, and married mates who were understanding—who did the home decorating, bought and chose outfits, and whose cooking they could rely on. Their partners may have even hidden the little "secret" so well that even their children don't know.

But times have changed. Women go to work and men eat out more often. Even "safe" jobs men held before now utilize color-coded computer generated information. Everybody is told to do his or her own thing. Even producers of consumer products have noted that some horrid color combinations have very enthusiastic male customers.

Retired couples often find that they suddenly fight about little odd things. It is often assumed that the arguments are due to spending so much time together, but often it can be due to CVC. The following situations are complaints I hear often from such couples. He insists on driving, but doesn't seem to stop for red lights or won't drive at night. She usually drove herself around, but now that he's insisting on doing the driving, she notices how bad a driver he is. He buys fruit, socks, and other items—all bargains she could do without because his choices are horrible. Other couples avoid them because color confusion comes across as cheating in board games. No one had ever challenged his color selections before (he probably hadn't made very many), and he is insulted at the insinuations of his argumentative and cheating behavior.

Another problem that can affect an older person with CVC is death of a spouse. If a wife has protected her husband most of his life by choosing his clothing, his foods, his decorations, and so on, so that no one would pick up on his CVC, in most cases he won't develop any skills to compensate. On the contrary, he will often become dependent on her. If she dies before him, he is left to dress himself, choose his own foods, figure out his own medications, decorate his own surroundings. At first his children or other friends may take his CVC as a form of grief—not caring about his own appearance or surroundings, or forgetting to take medication, or worse, taking the wrong medication. The color vision confusion he has experienced his whole life can now become a major stumbling block, and coupled with any other vision problems he acquires as he ages, eventually this can be misconstrued as senility. And, what's more, if no one has ever mentioned this problem before, these poor older people may actually begin to believe that they are senile.

This is the most difficult time of life to begin to learn where color cues are missed, and how to compensate for this, but it can be done. Labels can be put on clothing, foods, and medications, a child or friend can accompany this senior on food shopping trips. Things can be placed in specific locations in his home, and a checklist of locations can be made up for those whose memory just isn't what it used to be. (For more helpful tips, see Chapter 11, Coping With Color Vision Confusion.)

People who have inherited color vision confusion and have managed to lead a normal life otherwise, are far brighter than most. Instead of being "a bit slow" they have managed to live a life in which they have had to speak two visual languages, so to speak, all the time. They have to constantly "translate" in their minds that which they see and that which they think they are expected to see. These people have managed to store enough cues mentally so that they can compensate for cues they cannot decipher.

IN CONCLUSION

The relationship between vision, learning, and the brain is very complex. The brain makes notations and remembers visual information, and adds its comments to the mental memory files in ways we cannot yet comprehend. Seeing seems to be so easy and expected that we take it for granted, but in fact, digesting what we see, even if it is done in a split second, is mental work.

But what is even more miraculous is that we also have coping mechanisms for emergencies. It helps to have advance knowledge of the problem and an understanding of the problem at hand, in order to take actions that will lead to sensible results.

It would help all the more if those who are personally affected by seeing the wrong colors, or by not seeing some colors at times, would speak up. Maybe then there would be more attention given to CVC and changes would take place to help people cope.

10

How Are Families Affected by CVC?

Color vision confusion doesn't only affect the person who has the condition. Because so little is widely known about it, and even less is understood about it by the general population, it also tends to have an impact on family members. How strong an impact it has depends on two main factors: first, whether or not the person and his or her family are aware of the CVC, and second, whether or not the family and person with CVC are willing to accept and deal with the condition.

Often, people do not realize the underlying cause of their family feuds. It is well-known in the field of psychology that people often argue due to issues that never come up in the actual argument. In such cases, the argument is just a symptom of another problem. But when arguments spring up over color, they seem petty. Some may assume that there is another underlying problem—jealousy, for example—that has nothing to do with vision, ignorant of the fact that an inability to see "eye to eye" may be due to arguments about color as well as sight, and insight. Sadly, few counselors or psychologists give any consideration to color vision confusion as a cause of family rifts or, at the very least, sharp exchanges of insults, sad arguments, and painful accusations.

The problem may bury itself even deeper, as seen in previous chapters, when it is not even suspected that a person is colorblind. Disagreements can spring up over "not seeing" certain things, which can be interpreted by a family member as carelessness or ignoring instructions. So that, now, the arguments are not even over color, it seems as if the problem might be one person trying to slight the other.

Feelings get hurt, and the symptom, the argument, is mistaken as the problem, when color vision confusion is at fault. Unfortunately, it is not likely that a family counselor will be able to figure out the vision problem.

WHEN A CHILD IS COLORBLIND

When a parent does not understand a child's colorblindness, and refuses to try, the psychological result to the child can be devastating. (Of course, parents refusing to try to understand any problem a child may have can be equally devastating.) As we read in the last chapter about the colorblind boy who refused to shoot targets with his father, such cases not only affect the child's sense of self-worth, but can often affect the marriage of the parents—these two divorced. (Fortunately, going through this with his parents helped him form a closer relationship with his own girlfriend.)

When children of any age are faced with a problem, and recognize that they don't have the support or understanding of their parents, they're in they unenviable position of having to learn to deal with it on their own. But that does not mean that they are truly alone. Children can call on other supportive individuals—such as other family members, school counselors, good friends, members of the clergy, pediatricians—in order to improve their coping skills. It certainly would be desirable for any of the people who are called upon by a child to have some understanding of CVC. But even if they don't, the situation is not hopeless. Children seem to instinctively know who is empathic, as well as who they can talk to. This book can be a good reference, giving additional insight and understanding to these compassionate people in their role of support.

Support should come from other sources as well, for instance, in school. In an earlier chapter we had mentioned the case of a young girl who was so overwhelmed by not being able to see colors that she started to refuse to open her eyes in school. She never played with other children and refused to go outdoors. She was placed in a class for the visually impaired, a "sight-saving" class. This made things worse. She was branded as uncooperative and was transferred to a state school for the feeble-minded. (Sadly, few school counselors are well-informed about the condition, even today.)

The parents could not cope with the thought of a "slow" child, and it put a heavy strain on their marriage. They divorced. But her mother had hope. It took years for her to get the girl out of the school for the feeble-minded. It turned out that the girl is one of those rare individuals who has total colorblindness. Her vision is monochromatic. Sadly, her family life was badly damaged.

Although teachers and administrators know that many children have difficulty within the educational system, they must keep their minds open to different explanations for these difficulties. CVC has been shown to be one of the obstacles to efficiency in learning, reading, and using the computer, among many other activities. Although most teachers and educational professionals are now trained to recognize subtle reactions from children to indicate a learning disability, it is hoped that they will become more aware of the particular interference caused by CVC, and participate in the development of more effective compensatory mechanisms for children experiencing these problems, as well as color vision tests.

WHEN A SPOUSE IS COLORBLIND

When a mate is colorblind, a big part of the manner in which it is handled, as with other cases, is whether or not it is known that the person has CVC. When it is known, most partners will come up with a system to make life a little easier—marking containers with colors that can be read easily, putting specific things in assigned places. But if it isn't known that one partner is colorblind, life can be very confusing. More confusion is added when colorblindness is acquired after marriage—from medication or an accident—and neither partner realizes that is has crept into their lives.

One story that was related to us illustrates this point very well. A woman said that her husband seemed to make constant mistakes when playing board games that involved color. He had never before cheated when playing games, and he had always had full color vision, so she couldn't figure out what was going on. She wondered if his mental capabilities were on the decline, or if he was reverting to his "second childhood," or if he was possibly in the early stages of Alzheimer's disease.

Only after she was asked whether he was on any medications, or was diabetic, or affected by any other problem that could medically explain his condition, did she realize that she was jumping to terrible conclusions. It was almost a relief to know that medication could have been the cause of her husband's color vision confusion, and that she had been imagining a far worse fate than the facts warranted. Wouldn't it have been better if she didn't have to worry so needlessly? Wouldn't it be good if doctors understood that such side effects as color vision confusion can be terribly confusing and worrying? With this understanding, they would make sure that all side effects were discussed when prescribing medications.

Another woman said that she had never considered the possibility that arguments with her husband were caused by a color vision problem. Unfortunately, we didn't sort through all of this and figure out the problem until after his death. She eventually realized that this was why he had seemed so attached to her. He would only go out at night if she drove. He would only develop photographs, a favorite hobby of his, when she was in the darkroom, because he could not see what was going on in the red light. He always needed her to pack his clothes for the many business trips he took as the accountant/vice president of a major company. There were many other times that he needed her help as well. Years after his death, she recalled that the navy had refused to take him, although he was a whiz in math, could calculate in his head, and had passed all the other tests he had been given. (He did serve in the army, from which he was honorably discharged.)

In his later years, he developed a heart condition. His wife explored different ways to keep his mind occupied. She encouraged him to take an art class. He was very interested in the class as long as he drew or copied things in tones of brown and black and white, the very tones that had been used to decorate their home. She tried to convince him that, instead of drawing things to suit the decor of the house, he should paint a picture that suited him. And so, he came home with a picture of a floral display of pink, white, khaki, and black flowers. When she asked him why he had not used happy colors, he replied that he had. To him, you see, black was probably equal to red, khaki was equal to orange or green, and white was equal to yellow, light blue, or pink. The pink might well have represented blue to him. He was hurt that she appeared not to like his picture, that she had said that she could not make any sense of it. So, he lied and told her that it was an abstract painting.

To force him out of this "morbid habit," as she called it, she bought him a set of pastels. However, he looked at the pastels, and stopped doing art work altogether. His wife did not realize that he could not tell one color from another in that box.

As she and I slowly untangled her recollections, she began to realize why her husband had wanted her involved in his photography hobby, in his darkroom, and in mixing the chemicals. He could not see in the red light that lit the room, could not mix the chemicals, nor tell if the developer was doing its job properly. The possibility of color confusion had never occurred to her before.

She also learned something about herself. She learned that it was not only her husband's death that kept her depressed, but the color scheme of the house. She had never before given any thought to it. She had a strong desire to make her husband happy and thus accepted his selections of home furnishings and decoration. She snapped out of her doldrums by redecorating her home.

A surprising number of women have lived a lifetime not knowing that their husbands were colorblind. In their opinions, the men had left the selection of socks, shirts, or ties to their wives because they knew "their women had good taste." The selection of curtains and interior decoration was "the women's department." The men tended to buy the cars. Today, name brands offer whole sets of housewares and outfits of clothing that are sure to match. They cost more but they do not require much color coordination.

When a problem such as CVC causes strain in a relationship—especially when it is not even known that CVC is the culprit—improving communication is essential if the partners want to remain together. In fact, in the examples you've just read, the main reason some marriages break up is not so much because of CVC, but because the partners are not able to unite in discussions to find out the source of their problems.

Couples dealing with "undiagnosed" problems need to be especially understanding and flexible. Rather than one partner thinking the other is "nuts," it is more important to try to figure out what is going on to cause odd behavior. These things need to be talked out. Each partner needs to look at the situation through the other person's eyes, try to empathize, and come up with a more constructive way of dealing with difficult situations.

Couples also have to learn how to listen. A person who is going through a problem—such as CVC—may be sharing some important information about his or her difficulties that would otherwise be overlooked by an impatient spouse. Partners with communication problems tend to make statements instead of asking questions. Questions such as "What are you seeing?" or "Can you describe to me why you've worn that article of clothing?" can elicit far more meaningful information in helping a couple work together to develop compensatory mechanisms than sarcastic questions such as "What were you thinking when you put *that* on?" or "Did you get dressed in the dark?"

The first step, however, is recognizing that better communication is needed. Unfortunately, some couples find out too late, or are so stubborn in their opinions that they never realize this at all.

WHEN A PARENT IS COLORBLIND

When both parents are colorblind, the whole topic may mean little to them. To them, their lives are "normal." But chances are, even in these cases, both parents and children could benefit from a better grasp of the problem.

Consider the case of Barbara. Family feuds regarding colors were part of Barbara's upbringing, as her father and his brother were partners in a furniture store. Both of them were colorblind but would not admit to it. Each month, when the window display had to be changed, the situation was very unnerving. Furthermore, her mother could hardly stand her father's tantrums when customers complained that the sofa delivered was the wrong color. To make matters worse, her mother was also colorblind. As you can well imagine, none of this was good for business!

Wild arguments filled Barbara's life. She could not determine who was right—since both her parents were colorblind, she was too (as hereditarily expected). She dreaded being asked to arbitrate or to suggest how the window display looked.

To make matters worse, too many fights about Barbara's "carelessness" had caused her own marriage to end in divorce. Her husband was tired of having his socks mismatched. She told him to take care of his own socks. He had walked out of the house one day with pants and jacket mismatched because she had hung the two items on one hanger. Of course, her sons had always been on their "mother's side" because they are colorblind as well. This angered her husband all the more. He left and refused to pay alimony or child support.

Lack of understanding about (or complete denial of) CVC is often, as seen here, the cause of frustration, which manifests into anger. Although anger is unpleasant, people in successful relationships deal with anger too, only more effectively. By trying to avoid these intense emotions, or pretending that there isn't a problem, nothing gets resolved. To successfully deal with anger and frustration, focus on the reasons for these frustrations—deal with the cause, not the symptom. What is really at issue? Even if the exact reasons cannot be pinpointed, the conversation is still being guided in a more positive direction. Use calming tones in conversation. This is far more productive than getting angry and lashing out.

OTHER RELATIONSHIPS AFFECTED BY CVC

Another woman, Renee, got some very revealing insight from watching her boyfriend deal with his colorblind sons. The two boys were forever bickering and accusing each other of cheating on board games. It turned out that both had color vision confusion, which was what was causing the arguments.

The father, who had normal color vision, began to re-examine why he had been having arguments with his first wife. It turned out she was colorblind, but he had never heard of a woman inheriting color vision confusion before. He had simply thought she was being contrary all the time, which was, to him, typical female behavior.

On discovering his attitude towards women, Renee decided that she was liable to have bigger arguments with this man than the boys were having with each other. She was sure she had done right by stepping away from that relationship.

One more case is worth noting. A nurse named Jennifer had been going out with a young architect who asked her to marry him. She was, however, very puzzled by him. She could not understand how someone so artistic could always pick such strange colors. She decided to marry him anyway, but nearly called the wedding off when he insisted on wearing a mint green tuxedo. He said it was a light grey and perfect for their afternoon wedding. She said it looked horrid and would rather have him wear black, but he refused to wear black in summer. A bargain was at last struck. He would wear white. But she was still uncomfortable. What would it look like, a bride in white and a groom in white?

"Let's make believe we are king and queen of vanilla" he said. It made her laugh, just as he had always found a way to make her laugh. When they said their vows no one knew why they could hardly restrain themselves from laughing. They laugh about it even now, thirteen years later, although he still makes her want to climb up a tree sometimes when it comes to colors.

As you can see, having a good sense of humor can be a very effective coping strategy. Jennifer and her architect were able to use humor to diffuse what might otherwise have been a very tense situation for them. When there is nothing you can do about a particular problem, being able to laugh at it can make the difference between coping and not coping. (You can find out more about using humor in difficult situations in Chapter 11, Coping With Color Vision Confusion.)

LIVING IN FEAR

Some people with CVC have learned that it is hard for the people you care about to judge you for your vision deficiency if they don't know about it. Jean is a Cajun thirty-two-year-old, twice-married, and he is colorblind. Most of the people he grew up with, in "Indian country," in North Carolina saw as he did, which is significant if you consider what these people did in the early years of this country, they made baskets. These people never considered that they were red/green colorblind, especially since his ancestors had prided themselves on being able to tell when the wild green grasses were ripe and what they would look like as they dried and were woven into baskets. Originally, these baskets were not only sold to tourists; they were used for holding catches of fish, hanging meats to dry from limbs of trees, collecting wild fruits and tubers, and even for steaming foods and medicines in the ancient tradition. These Native Americans only needed to recognize the shades of the grasses to know that they were ready for gathering—not too much room for error when everything registers as a type of brown, but the focus is on textures.

This type of selective vision was very important in centuries gone by for Native Americans. But Jean was not weaving any baskets. In fact, his family never had. (His maternal grandfather had been a school principal.) Jean was a gentle soul, a man with appealing looks, and a strong sense of responsibility. He was also bright, but for some reason he had never gotten very far. He had been a carpenter for years and could tell the shades and textures of wood at a glance. But somehow he fumbled when it came to dealing with electrical tools. It caused him to be slow. It caused him to lose jobs, which, in turn, caused him to lose his first wife (who has custody of their children).

When the local community college offered a program in industrial construction management, a funded program that was free to students, he signed up. The course in electrical work was out of the question as far as he was concerned, as was the course that focused on the make-up of industrial chemicals. Why? Because he never got the colors right.

Jean experienced much silent pain. He was terrified of arguments with his second wife. She would get annoyed that he could not match socks or pass an exam in electronics. She wanted him to "grow up" and stop trying to "look for attention." He was worried about a second divorce.

In the past, he had been unable to explain his behavior. As he became knowledgeable about his CVC, his behavior seemed to make more sense to him. He could face himself better. He also realized that he could work in industrial electrical management, as long as he could hire people to do the wiring for him. And, just as importantly, his wife is learning to understand the stress caused by his color confusion. She now knows that it was not simply silly behavior.

IN CONCLUSION

Jean's story points out the importance of feeling good about who you are (regardless of CVC). Self-esteem is one of life's most precious commodities. Those who like themselves invariably do better for themselves and live happier lives than those who don't. Surveys of individuals with a variety of medical disorders clearly show that self-esteem does not have to be directly related to the existence of these disorders. In other words, you can like yourself, even if you have CVC! (This will seem like an unnecessary statement only to those with good self-esteem.)

Focus on the good things about yourself, regardless of how CVC is affecting you. You are not a CVC victim, you are a person who happens to have CVC. Regardless of how the condition affects you, you are still a good, productive person. And, the better you deal with CVC, the better you'll feel about yourself, and the less silent pain you'll experience.

11

Coping With Color Vision Confusion

If there is any group that has allowed itself to be sold short, it is the group of people that has color vision confusion. Most people with CVC have, out of necessity, accepted (with humor) the unusual world in which they live. Recognizing that "what you see is what you see," most individuals with color vision confusion try to go on with their lives as normally as they can. But this is a daily struggle. They continually have to translate or interpret what they see in order to conform to what they think others see or expect them to see. People with color vision confusion also have to consider whether what they do or say will be accepted by others; after all, they can hardly explain to others the differences in what they see.

No one has, as yet, developed a way to correct color vision confusion, but many who were born with the condition consider it to be a unique experience. Like many people who have lived their entire lives with a physical impairment or disability, many with CVC would rather remain as they are, although no one knows how they would react if they could see what they are missing. Certainly, they would have to relearn many visual cues.

For the present, whether you have color vision confusion or live with someone who has it, your goal is to learn to live with it better. As you've probably realized by now, living successfully with any kind of a problem involves three important steps:

1. Understanding as much as you can about the problem.
2. Making any changes that are feasible to make your life more com-

fortable and efficient.

3. Learning to cope more successfully with anything that you cannot change.

With regard to these three steps, hopefully, this book has given you a greater understanding of CVC, as well as informing you of current efforts to research color vision confusion. There are always things that can be done to improve the ability to better live with, and compensate for, CVC (see Helping Yourself Day to Day on page 145). Throughout the book, you have gained insight and information about many of the things you can do to more effectively deal with and enhance your life with CVC. But what about the things that you cannot change? That's where coping with stress and anxiety comes in. There are wonderful coping strategies that can help you deal with the reality you cannot change. So let's move on to the third step and talk about some of the helpful strategies.

PINPOINT YOUR CVC CONCERNS

The first step in improving your coping ability is to determine exactly what areas need better coping! This may sound simple, but doesn't it make sense? What are the ways that CVC affects you? What hurdles continue to cause stress and trouble you? What have you tried to do about them? What factors cannot be changed? The answers to these questions will get you started in pinpointing the CVC-related concerns that you want to cope with better.

Once you have identified areas for improvement, you will want to start selecting strategies that can help you. This chapter will discuss strategies falling into six important areas: using relaxation techniques, benefiting from a sense of humor, improving your thinking, enhancing your support system, attending (or forming) support groups, and considering professional help.

RELAXATION PROCEDURES

Using relaxation techniques regularly can be an important part of your efforts to better handle CVC. They are important for two reasons:

1. To reduce the physiological and psychological impact of any symptoms (either physical or emotional) you are experiencing.

HELPING YOURSELF DAY-TO-DAY

Although color is a major cue that most people rely on for object recognition, there are other ways of recognizing and coordinating different things. Following is a list of various "tricks" or compensatory mechanisms that people with CVC have used successfully in the past, and that, hopefully, will work for you.

• Buy appliances with green, amber, or white lights and digital information on them. You may also want to request that such appliances or equipment be used at work if new purchases are being made.

• Focus on contrasts of textural effects in clothing and interior decor, they are as interesting as colors. The same goes for computer-generated charts.

• When conservative dress is a must, make sure that the suit is a solid color and the tie is a pattern or stripe as a counterpoint. You might also want to get a pocket handkerchief to match your tie if you feel the solid color suit looks too funereal.

• Keep a coordinated tie in the pocket of your suit jacket when you hang it up for the next wearing. Or, keep the belt to a dress on the same hanger. You can also use permanent ink to write on the inside of belts to help match them up with coordinating clothing.

• Tack a small piece of suit fabric to the back of a tie to remind you which suits it goes with.

• When decorating a room, look for coordinated sets. You might also ask a salesperson to put together a set like the one the store has on display, if it is not too expensive.

• Keep a marking pen of a color that you can distinguish clearly on hand at all times, including in the car. (We suggest you try brown, violet, orange, or blue.) This way, if you have to ask for directions, you can request that the person also highlight your map.

• Make sure pills are in clearly labeled bottles, or else in containers with specific numbers on them. The same goes for anything that will be put away in a container other than its own—food, chemical cleaners, beverages, etc.

• Colorblind children often enjoy scented crayons. Crayola makes colors to coincide with the smells of fruits of the same color and other interesting and appealing smells. For more information, call 1-800-CRAYOLA.

• Let your colorblind child select the style of clothing he or she wants to wear, and then follow-up by selecting the rest of the outfit to match the child's selection. This allows the child to have a say in what he or she wears, and prevents tantrums. Discuss in advance which items the child will be allowed to pick, and which items you will pick.

• Learn to associate things with their scents and sounds, not just their colors. The more sophisticated the society, the more we tend to lose the value of

distinguishing by scent and sound. Revive the delicate use of these senses, you may find this of value in situations you never before imagined.

• *You already know that you cannot expect people to understand how you see, but there is a simplified way to explain it. Ask if they have ever watched a black and white movie or television. Do they envision colors while they watch? Do they wish they knew what the real color of that actress's hair, or the dress she is wearing? To further clarify, remind them that you see colors that seem to be different from the ones they see—like a television whose colors are adjusted wrong—and this causes visual confusion.*

• *Allow for the topic to be aired. Don't hide it as a private "secret." Once upon a time people hushed up the need for hearing aids, glasses, and left-handed scissors. Let it be known that there are no such tools to aid people with CVC.*

• *Send a copy of this book to anyone who does not seem to understand that you have a sharp mind, and fine vision, but your color vision is confused. Remember that if you share your ways of coping with others, you will be offering the world some very valuable advice. And, if others understand why you need to cope differently, people may well admire your ability to cope as you do.*

2. To eliminate or control any situations, circumstances, or stressors that may make it even more difficult for you to handle CVC

Relaxation techniques can be used in two important ways: preventively and curatively. What does this mean? Preventive use of the techniques gets your body used to them and the way they work, and builds up your confidence in them before the problem occurs. This reduces the likelihood of extreme stress responses. Curative use of the techniques refers to your using the techniques to maintain or regain control at the first sign of, or after a problem has arisen.

Why do relaxation techniques work? Because as relaxation increases, tension dissipates, which is the ultimate goal of the techniques. Learning how to respond to an anxiety-provoking situation with a relaxation technique will reduce the intensity of the anxious feeling. (And in the case of preventive techniques, can lessen the initial tension response.)

It is important to practice relaxation techniques as frequently as you can. The more you practice, the more your body will become conditioned to these more comfortable, healthy feelings, and the more quickly you will benefit from them.

There are a number of different types of relaxation techniques that can help you. Here are three effective techniques that are easy to learn: calming breathing, progressive relaxation, and brief relaxation.

Calming Breathing

Practice calming breathing to reduce stress when you are relatively calm. Recline or lie down on a bed, breathing slowly and leisurely in a way in which you can feel yourself becoming relaxed. When you inhale, fill your lungs and hold your breath for just a fraction of a second before exhaling. Breathe in gently and slowly. Breathe in a normal amount of air, filling the lower part of your lungs. Then breathe out easily and normally. Not every breath has to be a deep breath. Under normal conditions, you will mix deep breaths with more shallow breaths. Try to use the same pattern in your calming breathing.

As you practice these deep breathing techniques, be sure that your breathing does not become too rapid. Breathing too deeply and rapidly can cause hyperventilation. Avoid this by breathing slowly and comfortably, even when you breathe deeply.

Progressive Relaxation

A technique that can help you to relax your muscles is called progressive relaxation. Think of all the muscles of the body as being divided into four groups: the muscles from the feet up to the trunk, the muscles of the trunk (including the abdomen, back, and chest), the muscles of the arms from the hands to the shoulders, and the muscles of the neck, face, and head. You can choose the sequence that you use in tensing and then relaxing these groups and the muscles in them.

To start, get yourself into a comfortable position for your uninterrupted practice session. Then tense each muscle or group of muscles, squeezing tightly (but not too tightly) for five to seven seconds. Then relax and feel the tension drain out of the muscle or muscle group.

After going through all the muscles at least once, picture a pleasant, relaxing scene while allowing relaxation in all muscles to deepen.

Brief Relaxation

Brief relaxation techniques are beneficial because you can use them anywhere, whenever you need them, to feel immediate results. They will help you to relax after something makes you tense. In addition, practice will make your body less vulnerable to anxiety.

One example of brief relaxation is the "Quick Release." Be sure you read the directions completely before beginning this procedure.

Close your eyes, take a breath and hold it. At the same time concentrate on as many muscles as possible, and tense them (without straining yourself). Hold your breath and keep your body tense for approximately six seconds. Then let your breath out in a whoosh and allow the tension to drain out of your body. Let your body go limp. Keep your eyes closed, and breathe rhythmically and comfortably for approximately twenty seconds. Repeat this six second/twenty second cycle two more times.

As you can see, this entire procedure takes less than two minutes. Initially, you should attempt to practice it at least five different times a day. In addition, any time you feel any anxiety and would like to control it, the "Quick Release" can help. Three repetitions are not always necessary. Sometimes one cycle is sufficient; at other times you may need more than the three recommended. You be the judge.

HAVE A GOOD SENSE OF HUMOR

Humor can be an effective way to deal with a problem. Whether it is hearing a joke from someone else, laughing at oneself, or creating one's own jokes, humor can be a very relaxing way of dealing with any day-to-day problems that occur because of CVC. Humor can be a distraction. Why is this important? When you are stressed, your emotions may keep you from thinking clearly. Humor can alleviate stress, and break the "hold" that stress has on you, allowing you to look at a given situation more clearly and determine a better way to respond. You may be able to look at your stressful situation more objectively, which can help you to handle it more effectively. As you can imagine, because of the difficulties that CVC can cause, you want to be able to control as many emotional responses to colorblindness as possible, so objectivity is an important goal.

The ability to laugh at oneself is a surprisingly helpful coping strategy, and puts others at ease as well. How well this works, however, depends on the extent of the problem. For example, it's just about impossible (and probably ridiculous) to laugh at oneself while going through a crisis. But we are sure there are some humorous things you can say or think of concerning CVC. Are you laughing already? Are you smiling, at least?

WORK ON YOUR THINKING

Many people with CVC handle it well, and are not adversely affected by it, because they are able to think appropriately, constructively, and realistically about the condition. Others may be having a much harder time because of their inability to control their thinking, and may have over-expectations that are unrealistic.

The difference between being happy and unhappy is not whether or not you experience negative thoughts. Rather, the difference is determined by how successful you are at dealing with any negative thoughts that you do have. Here are a few suggestions for working on your thinking.

Reword Your Negative Thoughts

If having CVC leads to any negative emotions, such as fear, anger, or depression, it is because of your thinking pattern. Therefore, it is important to work on constructive techniques to change the way you think. For example, you may want to learn how to restructure (or reword) negative thoughts by turning negatives into realistic positives. This is called "cognitive restructuring." Identify and reword your negative thinking. Replace words that are inappropriate and counterproductive with more positive and realistic ones. For example, you might think "My life is horrible because of my color vision confusion." Using this example, you might change your words to think "I may not be happy about CVC, but should I really say that my whole life is horrible? Aren't there some things about my life that I'm happy about? Let me focus on them." This helps you to do two things. First, it teaches you to recognize the negative or inappropriate thoughts that are making it hard for you. Second, by rewording these thoughts into more realistic, positive ones, you will improve the way you deal with problems and emotions.

Think Clearly and Positively

The quality of your thoughts can help you to feel better, even if you can't change anything going on around you. Try, for example, to use the present tense when framing your thoughts. You will want your spoken words and inner expressions to be positive. Try to avoid terms that are extreme negatives such as "useless," "tragic," "can't," "impossible," etc. If your thoughts are not clear and concise, STOP! Begin again. Once you recognize clear, positive thoughts, write them down. Read them over. Continue using and repeating this process. You may never see a rainbow, but think of that pot of gold on the other side that nobody has yet found, not even those with full color vision.

Use Positive Affirmations

A positive affirmation is a positively worded statement about yourself that you either say out loud or think to yourself. Repeat this positive statement as frequently as you realistically can. Why do this? The more you repeat positive thoughts to yourself, the more you will start to believe them. Don't be put off if, at first, you don't. As long as your affirmations are realistic, this technique can work for you.

Avoid Comparisons With Those Who Have Normal Vision

Now and then, those with CVC unhappily compare themselves to others who don't have it. But this is counterproductive. If you are in an emotionally fragile state and you do this, you will tend to "fall short" in contrast with the positives of those around you. Why do that? You can compare yourself with any person with regard to any characteristics. There will always be people who are better than you, as well as people who are worse than you, no matter what their characteristics are. Remind yourself of this when you find yourself automatically getting into comparisons. Use this as a reason not to continue the comparison. Just concentrate on being who you are.

IMPROVE YOUR SUPPORT SYSTEM

Nobody likes problems. But it can be much easier to deal with any kind of problem if you have supportive people, family or friends, behind you. All too often, relationships break down because of a lack of understanding or a lack of communication. Let's discuss two ways of improving your relationships—educating others and improving communication with them.

Provide Education

Although CVC may not seem like a major medical disorder requiring sig-

---

CVC IN HIGH PLACES

If it seems to you that color vision confusion is a road block to success, then take into consideration the two candidates who ran for the office of United States President in 1996. President Bill Clinton, running for re-election, and Senator Bob Dole, from Kansas, both have inherited red/green color vision confusion.

For the televised debates that took place before the election, a system had to be devised for letting the candidates know when they were on camera, and how much time they had to speak, without resorting to colored lights. According to Jim Lehrer of PBS, who was chosen as moderator of the debates because of his reputation for fairness and distaste for sensationalism, a system of three lights was used. When the first light came on, the candidate knew he had 30 seconds on camera. When the second light came on, he knew he had 15 seconds left. The third light signaled his camera time was up.

---

nificant intervention, it still can have an impact on the person with the condition, as well as others who have relationships with you. It can especially be problematic for family members (as seen in the previous chapter).

All too often, a major reason for these problems is the lack of knowledge or understanding of CVC. Sit down and talk with those individuals who can't seem to understand what you are going through. You should have two main goals:

1. First, try to provide additional education about CVC (this book can certainly help!), with the goal of making them more sensitive to how CVC affects you. (Anticipate, though, that if they have had difficulty understanding CVC before this, not much may change). Ideally, you would like them to "walk a mile in your shoes." For example, suggest that they wear glasses with colored filters for an entire day. They will see how colored filters can distort the colors of the most commonly perceived objects. Explain your own personal cues and how you make sense of what you see. It may be an eye-opener for others.

2. If you can't change their understanding, attitude, or support, at least request that they give you space to deal with CVC in ways that are best for you. For example, if you have trouble coordinating the

colors of you clothing, instead of being critical or giving you a hard time, let them either help you, or not say anything that might be counterproductive.

Improve Communication

Good communication is the key to good interpersonal relationships. Often, relationship cohesiveness is adversely affected when lines of communication break down. An essential way to improve strained relationships is to improve communication. If you are having difficulty living day-to-day with your CVC, this can be helped by discussing this with those significant people in your life. Let's discuss a few suggestions for improving communication with those who are important to you.

Many communication problems occur because the message you want to deliver is not being verbalized in a helpful way. Others may be offended by inappropriately-worded statements. So think before you speak. Phrase comments constructively. It would not be helpful to angrily say, "I can't stand the fact that you have no idea what I'm going through." Say things the way you would want to hear them from others. For example, it would be better to say, "It's probably impossible for you to totally understand how CVC can be a problem. How about if I try to explain it to you?" This can make others more receptive to what you have to say.

Be a better listener. Being a better listener leads to being a better communicator. Try to ask others the way they feel about the issue. Don't interrupt when people are expressing their feelings or opinions. Be sure you are fully aware of what they are saying. You may even want to restate their comment in your own words to show that you understand what they just said. This will also give them an idea as to how you would like them to listen to you in the future. Speaking openly about the condition will help them understand, and it will help you feel better too.

ATTEND (OR FORM) SUPPORT GROUPS

Self-help or support groups can be very helpful for many different medical problems. Although, at the present time, there is no group specifically for CVC, there may be groups with similar interests that can be helpful. Consider the following suggestions:

- Check with other people you know who have CVC to find out if they know of any helpful groups.
- Check with other people you know who have any visual problems to find out if they are aware of any groups to consider.
- Check the telephone book, and talk to your physician or local hospital to find organizations that might sponsor relevant support groups.
- Contact a local branch of the American Self-Help Clearinghouse, an organization that has a directory of all self-help or support groups in the country (201-625-7101). In this way, you will find out if there are any groups that focus on CVC or similar problems.
- Get on the Internet and start snooping around for any chat groups that may talk about CVC or vision problems. The Achromatopsia Network has a home page that invites those with this rare disorder, as well as those with light sensitivity and CVC to become "Friends of the Achromatopsia Network." Or, you may just find one other person who has some information that may help you with a specific problem. Either way, this is a form of support group.

If you still have not found a group that interests you, you might want to get involved in forming one. Here are some suggestions that you can use if you are interested in trying to form a CVC support group:

- Speak to a representative of the American Self-Help Clearinghouse. Request information about starting a group for people with CVC. This organization has wonderful materials that can help you begin this process.
- Set up a tentative, convenient time (e.g., evening or weekend) and place (e.g., local library, hospital, or church) for an "organizational" meeting.
- Once you have established a first date and place, contact anyone in your area who may be aware of others with CVC (for example, contacting eye doctors or opticians might be a good way to start).
- Post notices for interested people to contact you to get additional information.

The benefits of setting up a support group would be well worth it. Members learn how others handle the problems of CVC. Groups provide a forum for the exchange of feelings and ideas, as well as suggestions on how to cope better. People with CVC can see that they are not alone. This is probably the most important reason for belonging to a group. Groups can be wonderful for family members too, giving family members the chance to get some support of their own.

CONSIDER PSYCHOLOGICAL COUNSELING

Although self-help procedures can be helpful for some individuals, there are many cases in which the best way to cope with CVC may be to work with a qualified professional who specializes in this area. (This is not intended to suggest that CVC can only be dealt with through professional services. However, it may be helpful for you to look for professionals available in your area.) Speak to your doctor, or another reputable source, to obtain the name of an expert in this area who understands the social stresses brought on by color vision confusion.

When might you want to speak to a professional? Psychological intervention may be necessary if difficulties dealing with color vision confusion are affecting you emotionally. For example, if you are depressed because you have lost your job due to the need for "normal" color vision, and nothing seems to help you to feel better, you might benefit from professional help. Or if you have stopped socializing totally because you are so frustrated about people making fun of your blunders, the aid of professional assistance might help.

There are many ways that professional treatment can be helpful, including learning how to better deal with your feelings, using strategies more effectively, and helping your family better understand what you are going through.

Get Help With Feelings

Being able to talk to somebody objective and supportive can be very reassuring. Professionals can help you to put your feelings into a more appropriate perspective. They can discuss different ways of looking at an issue that you may have only been considering in one, emotionally unpleasant way. Professionals can help you learn effective coping strategies to deal with any problems you may face. For example, an understanding professional can offer ideas for different actions you can take, or different ways of thinking about things you can't change and sort out possible steps you can take to ease your path in life.

Get Help With Techniques

The therapeutic techniques the professional would use really depend on what emotional reaction or problem needs improvement. For example, if you fear how others are going to deal with your CVC, a therapist may feel that it is helpful to work with a procedure called systematic desensitization. What is systematic desensitization? If you feel anxious, it is because you have become sensitive to a particular stimulus or trigger. This is called sensitization. You have learned to be sensitized, and you can unlearn it as well, which is called desensitization.

The goal of systematic desensitization is to sever the connection between the trigger and your anxious response by replacing the anxious response with a more relaxed one. The professional will help you to achieve a deep level of relaxation, and then have you imagine the triggers that make you anxious, alternating them with relaxing imagery, until you are able to more comfortably imagine the previously anxiety-provoking triggers. Research has shown that this will enable you to actually experience the situation in real life with much less anxiety.

If your thinking is causing you problems, but you are not able to consistently change it on your own, a professional can help you. Cognitive techniques, for example, techniques that teach you how to reduce your negativity and use more realistically positive words, can be a useful therapeutic tool.

Although going into detail about techniques of this nature is beyond the scope of this book, suggested readings are listed in the appendix for further information.

Get Help With Family

Counseling can also be helpful in working with family members. By pointing out the emotional needs of someone with this silent burden, professionals can improve family unity and support. Of course, therapists themselves need to have a good grasp of the potential difficulties encountered because of CVC.

OPEN COMMUNICATION WITH YOUR EMPLOYER OR TEACHER

Having and keeping a job is very important. Remember that the

Americans with Disabilities Act assures people working conditions that will enhance job performance. Most people with CVC do not consider themselves disabled, but in this color-coded, computer-generated-information world, it would be wise to speak up and request color selections that make your job easier. Such changes have already been made in some places. However, this may require the education of the employer.

Consider the case of a house painter who is colorblind. You have to be sure this person knows the number of the color on the chart produced by the paint manufacturer in order to complete the job properly. In fact, colorblind painters are often much more meticulous and neat. They can often detect missed spots and wet spots better than painters with full color vision.

But, if you ask a colorblind lawyer to deal with charts or proofs for a case on a computer, or require a colorblind mechanic to figure out a printout of a computer test with no consideration for which colors should be used for codes, you are asking for the impossible. Even an excellent mechanic might be at a loss, and by asking for a translation he may open himself to doubt, ridicule, and lost time on the job.

If, however, the employer understands the facts regarding CVC, and the employee can be free to speak about it without fearing ridicule or the loss of his or her job, a different system of color-coding might be put in place. For instance, your employer may purchase specialized software, like Colorblind by Color Solutions, that allows perfect color reproductions for printers. Or, that particular aspect of the job might even be able to be relegated to someone else. Solutions can be as simple as that, and can benefit both employer and faithful employee.

IN CONCLUSION

There are many ways in which a person with CVC, as well as his or her family members, can be affected by the condition. As part of a well-rounded approach to proceeding through life in a happy, healthy, and productive way, it is important to focus on the whole problem. So, in addition to understanding CVC and its effects, learning how to cope with it as successfully as possible is a key to a good quality of life.

Conclusion

As yet, there is no known cure or corrective device for colorblindness. We are sure, by now, that this question has popped into your mind. However, being affected by CVC, you may have heard through various sources that there are methods in the works that may one day be used to correct CVC, or you may even have heard that they can already be used.

IN THE FUTURE

Scientists have made some effort to find devices, strategies, and approaches that can be used to enable people with CVC to live more comfortably. Among the items being investigated are special lenses and lens implants to aid those who are already living with CVC; better use of color for coding in the home and office environments; genetic engineering that may one day prevent CVC; and methods are being explored to overcome the various obstacles encountered in the field of education, as well as beginning to teach students with CVC various coping skills to help them through life's obstacles. We have covered some of the methods being researched, so that you may see what has been accomplished, and possibly watch for them in the future.

Lenses

Although lenses have been, and still are, under investigation as a means of improving CVC, it is very unlikely that any one lens is going to satisfactorily resolve the problem. For example, there is a red lens that was developed by Rhode Island ophthalmologist Dr. Harry I. Zeltzer in 1974. Originally called the X Chrom lens, it enables a color-blind person to distinguish shades of red not seen before, although it makes shades of green appear darker. But it is difficult for people with CVC to explain what it is that they see.

Do the lenses help? Not for extended use. Research has suggested that the X Chrom lens has limited use. Even Dr. Zeltzer has cautioned that this lens is not useful to all colorblind people. For one thing, it can be used only in one eye at a time. It makes that eye look bloodshot. What's more, not all colors become clearer. In fact, it has found an unexpected use by gamblers in casinos, where bloodshot eyes are the norm, by enabling them to spot marked cards. The lenses have also been used by those who need to focus for limited periods on details, as in the design of textiles. So this device is not a solution to color-blindness.

For those rare case of achromatopsia, a special contact lens is being developed by the Wohlk Company of Germany under the name of Hydrolex. This lens has a centrally tinted area with the capacity to absorb 80 percent of the light that would normally filter through to the eye. This may be commercially available soon.

Lens Implants

Some people who have had lens implants after a cornea operation—who have always had full color vision—report seeing colors of far more saturated brilliance than before. Even those whose color vision had been well-developed have described astounding and fascinating changes in the manner in which they see colors. But it is also true that some colors, such as beige, seemed to become far less attractive.

It is not uncommon to hear those with lens implants swoon over the color of fire, which they see as a vibrant and brilliant violet with tones of sparkling cobalt blue. This is the same reaction these people have towards the color of the sky at dawn. Lightning has been said to be seen as the color violet in overwhelming intensity. Flowers radiate with colors. Asphalt looks like a bluer black. In fact, people who have lens implants often speak as if in awe—ecstatic and almost lyrical about the new color sight that they experience.

One description from a man who had a lens implant in 1987 is of particular interest. A practicing ophthalmologist, he had a new lens to correct cataracts in one eye, but not in the other. He spoke of seeing the flame of the gas jet as a brilliant blue with his "new eye" and a boring grey-green-blue color with the other. The new eye saw the saturation of red at sunset more vividly, and porcelain looked like a brilliant violet-white, while it looked simply white to the other eye. Greens seemed to be bluer and blues seemed to be leaning more toward purple. Although he found it a bit disconcerting to have such varied input, he preferred that to resigning himself to the information he had received from his original eye.

Can lens implants help if the basic problem is with inherited faulty cones? It's too soon to tell. There are some reports of improved and enhanced color vision as a result of lens implant surgery. Much more research is necessary. What kinds of lenses should be implanted? What colors can be better seen by those with CVC after implantation? Will all types of color confusion be helped by implants? These and many other questions need to be answered. Hopefully, the ongoing research will answer those questions.

Vitamin A

As mentioned in an earlier chapter, vitamin A plays a significant role in vision. But does it help those with color vision confusion? This question has often been asked. The unfortunate answer is that no one who was born with color vision confusion has ever reported gaining color vision by supplementing with vitamin A.

Vitamin A has been known to be important for good vision since 1917 when biologist George Wald of Harvard found the connection. Professor Wald found that vitamin A affects the retina, and we know that the retina is where the cones are, which allow for color vision. From that time on, it became fashionable for mothers to give their children cod liver oil, in part because it is rich in vitamin A. Today, we recognize many sources of vitamin A and its precursor, beta-carotene, so there is no need to ingest spoonfuls of oil. Instead, we can eat beef and chicken liver, eggs, and dairy products for vitamin A, or green and yellow-orange vegetables for beta-carotene.

But remember, those who have inherited color vision loss or confusion have missing or defective cones. Most often, those who acquire color vision loss have nerve damage rather than retinal damage, or are exhibiting some type of reaction to medications.

So despite research on the use of vitamin A, it has been concluded that no amount of vitamin A will restore damaged or absent color vision, whether the person was born with CVC or became colorblind for any of the various other reasons.

Genetic Engineering

Some hope that one day genetic engineering, or DNA manipulation, will allow us to wipe out CVC and many more harmful genetic conditions. More and more research is focusing on the burgeoning developments in the field of genetics. Although controversial, gene therapy, now being researched and developed for many different purposes, may soon be widely used for medical reasons. But what exactly is genetic engineering?

There are more than 4,000 known problems that are genetic in nature—that a person inherits either from his or her father, mother, or both. Genetic engineering attempts to manipulate the genes that pass on these "defective" traits. For example, in some cases missing genes can be added, or genes can be altered to retard the development of misformed organs. In some cases, defective genes can be eliminated.

The procedures involved with, and the results from, genetic engineering have varied. In some cases, genetic material is extracted from the patient, altered in the test tube, and then reintroduced with hopes that it will "take." In other cases, lasers have been used to "zap" genes into changing, mutating them in a sense. But genes are microscopic in size, and not all functions of all the genes have, as yet, been discovered. Humans have an amazingly intricate combination of genes. The ongoing Human Genome Project is attempting to identify all the genes and discover what they do. All of this work is very new.

The first successful attempt at genetic engineering took place only twenty years ago, and it was not done on humans. It took years before it was attempted on humans. Now it is starting to become more commonplace, but it still has not been used with regard to sight. In fact, genetic engineering is so new, so experimental, that top priority is still given to finding solutions for far more serious gene-related problems.

Perhaps genetic engineering will someday play a part in enabling persons to gain the full spectrum of color vision. But, CVC is not a priority in this field at this time.

Education

Techniques are being explored to modify and improve the education of those who are colorblind. This may be a useful adjunct to traditional education. Enabling individuals with CVC to learn effective compensation techniques may be a useful way of improving life functioning.

One example of strategic education was developed by the Japanese. They claim that they have a method of teaching people who are colorblind to recognize colors. However, "students" of this method have to return to school every six months or so. At this time, we are not sure exactly what is being taught to these students. In all probability, they are being taught to memorize certain ways of handling machinery, or reading certain codes on computers. The Japanese system has not been proved to be reliable.

Better Use of Color

As we learn more about the importance of color vision, as well as how color vision confusion can interfere with the quality of life, better use of color must be considered to be an important treatment approach to CVC. What particular color is seen does matter. How color is used does matter. After all, when a color is a primary carrier of information and the color is confused or is not seen, the transfer of information is severely restricted.

There are a number of ways that color can be used more efficiently. Applications of color coding may have to be reconsidered. For example, the color of many fire trucks and ambulances have already been changed. Think about it—when was the last time you saw an ambulance with red writing? It is more often blue and orange now.

Why the change? Dr. Stephen Solomon, an optometrist and volunteer fireman from Oswego, New York, who is a consultant to the National Firemen's Organization, states that using the new colors has dramatically cut down on accidents involving these vehicles while in transit responding to emergency calls. It has been found that yellow-green fire trucks can be seen by more people, more clearly than red ones, in all types of weather. And yet, even this color application needs further study.

In some theaters, the color of exit signs has already been changed from red to green. At least they can be seen in the dark by all.

Many road signs, construction hard hats, and other emergency gear is now colored orange, rather than red or yellow. This is also true of lights that indicate whether electrical tools or and appliances are on or off.

In Canada, recent research to aid those with color vision problems has led to traffic lights with a metal plate placed over them with a shape cut out for the light to shine through—a horizontal pattern for GO and a vertical for STOP. This is not unlike the diagonal pattern that was long ago included at railroad crossings. The Canadian system has proved successful and is being tried elsewhere, including several cities in the U.S., but no results are in yet. The problem with getting the results in the United States is that traffic signals are controlled individually in each town or city, so we can't make the change nationwide. And most of the time, when the grids are installed, the local citizens are not informed in any public manner as to why there are suddenly patterns over the traffic lights. Worse yet, the grids are often added in reverse designs. It tends to add more confusion than it prevents when there is no explanation of what they are for.

UNTIL CVC CAN BE CORRECTED. . .

Our society needs to become more attuned to the problem of CVC. Many more designs and elements that attract the senses, like motion and sound, need to be incorporated into non-verbal communication. Consider how the frequency of accidents at railroad crossings was cut down by introducing the diagonal design on the signs a century ago. Remember, too, that the international pictorial signs now in common use have proved to be of value. They can be effective regardless of linguistic barriers or levels of literacy. The issue of effective visual-communication is, thankfully, now being studied very seriously.

In 1994, the Commission International De L'Eclairage, an international commission that sets the standards for degrees of variation of industrial tints and names, decided to publish a report on color vision confusion and to offer suggestions for taking the matter into consideration when planning signals for visual information. This commission, known as CIE for short, is based in Vienna, Austria.

According to Dr. Janos Schanda, executive director of CIE, commission members will discuss color vision anbormalities during discussions of the importance of luminance, brightness, and clear communication in visual display units. Such units are often needed when international communication can be best achieved by visual rather than linguistic means. These discussions reveal a new awareness that there may be many more colorblind people than those responsible for graphic information had realized.

Another exciting bit of news is the development of an instrument that will help in measuring degrees of color vision accuracy. The instrument is currently being constructed by a graduate student in electro-optics engineering at Ben Gurion University in Israel. The project director is Dr. Chaim Lotem, who has a personal interest in the subject, as he is colorblind.

Some additional research in that direction is now being done by Michael Wogalter at the Renssalaer Polytechnic Institute. He is also working on incorporating sound into warning signals. Much more can be done. Much more will be done if people acknowledge the need for such efforts.

IN CONCLUSION

Well, you've just about finished this book. We've covered a lot of information about CVC. Progress has been made in understanding the problem, but this is only a start. Ongoing research continues to explore ways of helping those with CVC, as well as further improving the quality of life for the person with CVC.

Perhaps by the time you read this, some drug or treatment may have proved itself to be successful in reducing the effects of CVC. It remains to be seen which new developments can improve life with CVC. But at least people are working on the problem.

As public awareness and sensitivity about colorblindness increases, those with the problem will find it easier to cope with the limitations imposed by color vision confusion. Needless to say, many people handle their condition very well already, either because that's their nature, or because they have developed their own effective compensatory strategies. Is that you? Do you have tricks or methods that you've found have been helpful in living comfortably with CVC? If so, we'd like to hear from you. We would also like to know at what point in your life you discovered your CVC, and under what conditions.

Please write to us in care of Avery Publishing Group, 120 Old Broadway, Garden City Park, NY 11040. Strategies that may be helpful to large numbers of people with CVC will be included (with appropriate credit given!) in future editions of this book.

If you have any comments, information you feel is important, or additional questions, feel free to write to us in care of the publisher. We'd be happy to hear from you. But for now, look brightly ahead, act proudly, and enjoy life as colorfully as you can!

Bibliography

Abery S; "An Optometrist With Color Defect"; Education; Wiley & Sons; Vol. 14, No.1; Feb, 1989.

Abramov I, Gordon J; "Color Appearance: On Seeing Red, or Yellow, or Green, or Blue"; Annual Review of Psychology; 451-485; 1994.

Aiken RG; "Drug Induced Color Vision Deficiencies From Side Effects to Clinical Pharmacology"; Docum Opthal Proc Ser. 33, 467-476; 1982.

Allen C; "Learning and Memory"; *Perceptual and Motor Skills Magazine*; Vol. 59(1) 263-266; Aug 1984.

Angier N; "New Clues to Vision: People Whose Glasses Must Be Rose-Colored"; *The New York Times* Medical Science Section C3; Nov 17, 1992.

Applebome P; "The Tangled U.S. Case of the Colorblind Airman"; *The New York Times*; p.1.; March 4, 1987.

Arthur C; "Message of the President of the United States"; Doc 24; US Senate; Congressional Record; US Printing Office; Washington DC; 1883.

Asimov I; *A Biographical New Guide to Science*; Basic Books; 1984.

Aubourg PR, Sack GH Jr, Moser HW; "Frequent Alteration of Visual Pigment Genes in Adrenoleukodystrophy"; *Amer. Journal of Human Genetics*; 42(3): 408-13; March, 1988.

Benjamin J, Press J, Maoz B, Belmaker RH; "Linkage of a Normal Personality Trait to the Color-Blindness Gene: Preliminary Evidence"; *Biological Psychology*; 581-583; 1993.

Berman R ed; *Nelson Textbook of Pediatrics* (14th edition); WB Saunders Co; Philadelphia PA; 1992.

Berninger T; "Using Argon Laser Blue Light Reduces Opthalmologists' Color Contrast Sensitivity"; 0; Vol 107; p 1453-1458; 1989.

Berry M; "Hitting a Colorblind Wall"; Health Special: *San Francisco Examiner*; p.1; Dec. 21, 1991.

Birren, F; *A Grammar of Color: A Treatise on the Color System Albert Munsell*; Van Nostrand Reinhold Co.; NY; 1969.

Birren, F; *Color Psychology and Color Therapy*; Van Nostrand Reinhold Co; NY; 1976.

Birren F; *Color: A Survey in Words and Pictures*; University Books; NY; 1963.

Birren F; *Light Color and Environment*; Nostrand Reinhold Co; NY; 1969.

Birren F; "Color and Human Response"; Proceedings of 10th Annual meeting of the Canadian Society for Color; 1982.

Borenstein M, Marks L; "Color Revisionism"; *Psychology Today*; Jan., 1982.

Booth, Barony; *Language of Graphics*; Harry Abrams and Sons, Inc.; NY; 1980.

Boynton, RM; *Human Color Vision*; Holt Reinhard and Winston; NY; 1979.

Bresnick G, Smith V, Pokorny J: "Autosomal Dominantly Inherited Macular Dystrophy With Preferential Short Wavelength Sensitive Cone Involvement"; *American Journal of Opthalmology*; 108:265-276; September, 1989.

Bresnick GH, Crawford J, Groo A; "Urine Testing Inaccuracies Among Diabetic Patients With Color Vision Deficiencies"; VII *Doc Opthalmol Proc*; Ser 39, 393-404; The Hague; 1989.

Byrum W, Porter R ed; *Companion Encyclopedia of the History of Medicine*; Routledge; NY; 1993.

Cambell J; *The Grammatical Man*; Simon and Schuster Inc; NY; 1982.

Cirlot JE; *A Dictionary of Symbols*; Philosophical Library; NY; 1962.

Cole G; *Facets of Light: Colors, Images and Things That Glow in the Dark*; Exploratorium; San Francisco, CA; 1980.

Collins M; *Colour Blindness*; Keagn Paul Trench Tauber Co. Ltd; London; 1925.

Cooper BA, Ward M, Gowland CA, Mc Intosh JM; "The Use of the Lanthony New Color Test in Determining Effects of Aging on Color Vision"; *Lancet*; 338:1338; Nov, 1991.

Coren S, Hakstian R; "Color Vision Screening Without the Use of Technical Equipment; Scale Development and Cross Validation"; *Perception and Psychophysics* Vol 43 115-120;1988.

Corsino BV; "Color Blindness and Rorscharch Responsiveness"; *Journal of Personality Assessment*; 49:5: 533-534.

Cronin-Golomb A, Sugiura R, Corkin S, Growdon JH; "Incomplete Acchromatopsia in Alzheimer's Disease; *Neurobiology of Aging*; Vol. 14; pp 471-477; 1993.

Cruz-Coke R; *Color Blindness: An Evolutionary Approach*; American Lecture Series; Charles Thomas; 1970.

Davidson SP, Myslinski NR; "Shade Selection by Color Vision Defective Dental Personnel"; *J Prosthet Dent*; 63:97-101; 1990.

De Bono E; *Newthink*; Basic Books; 1967.

De Vreese LP; "Two Systems of Colour Naming Defects: Verbal Disconnection vs Colour Imagry Defect"; *Neuropsychologia*; Vol. 29 No. 1; pp 1-18; 1991

Dictionary of Organic Compounds; Vol 5; Chapman Hill; London 1982.

Directory of Agencies Serving the Visually Handicapped in the US; 22nd edition; American Foundation for the Blind; New York; 1984.

Dowling JE; *The Retina*; The Belknap Press of Harvard University Press; Cambridge MA; 1987.

Edwards I; "Fundamentals of Lighting"; *Optics and Photonics News*; 17-20;

Nov, 1996.

Eiseman L; *Alive with Color*; Acropolis Books; 1984.

Ekert M, Bujger Z, Cervoski B; "Early Detection of Inborn Dyschromatopsia in Preschool and Young Schoolchildren"; *Opthalomogia*; 209.

Encyclopedic Dictionary of Physics; J.L. Thewlis, editor-in-chief; Pergamon Press; Oxford England; 1962.

Engelking E; "Uber den verlauf der Richtverkurven bei den Anomalen Trichomaten"; *Klinikal Monatblat Augenheilt*; 78; 208-219; Berlin; 1927.

Farnsworth D; "The Farnsworth-Munsell 100 hue and dichrotomous tests for color vision"; *Journal of Optical Society of America*; 33, 568-578; 1943.

Farnsworth D; *The Farnwsorth Dichromous Test for Color Blindness*; Psych. Corp; NY; 1947.

Feher E, Myer K; "Children's Conceptions of Color"; Journal of Research in Science Teaching; 29/5 505-520; May 20, 1992.

Fletcher R, Yoke J; *Defective Colour Vision: Fundamentals, diagnosis and management*; A. Hilger, Boston; 1985.

Foster DH; *Inherited and Acquired Color Vision Deficiencies: Fundamental Aspects and Clinical Studies*; CRC Press, Boca Raton, FL; 1991.

Freeman L, Costa L; "Pure Alexia and Right Hemiachromatopsia in Posterior Dementia"; *Journal of Neurosurgery and Psychiatry*; 55:500-502; 1992.

Fuchs T; *Stage Lighting*; Benjamin Blom; NY; 1963.

Garmet C; *Light and Sight*; Aberland-Schuman; London; 1963.

Gobba F, Gallasi C, Imbriani M, Ghittori S, Candella S, Cavalleri A; "Acquired Dischromatopsia Among Styrene-Exposed Workers"; *Journal of Occupational Medicine*; Vol 33 No 7; July, 1991.

Gillon P, Gobba F, Cavallieri A; "Kinetics of Urinary Excretion and Affects on Colour Vision After Exposure to Styrene"; *Catedra di Medicina de Lavorno*; Universita di Modena Italy; vol 127:79-88; 1993.

Goethe W; *Theory of Colors*; MIT Press; Cambridge Ma; 1982 (reprint from 1840).

Granville W; "Colors Do Look Different After Lens Implant!"; *Color Research and Applications*; Vol 15, No1 59-61; Feb 1990.

Graphics Times; Megatek Corporation; San Diego, Ca; August, 1983.

Green E; "Two Criteria for the Selection of Color Vision Test Plates"; *Journal of the Optical Society of America*; Vol 35; Nov, 1945.

Grissom G; *A Volume of People*; Hawthorne Books Inc; NYC, 1957.

Hackman; "Color Vision Testing for the U.S. Naval Academy"; *Military Medicine*; 651-657; Dec, 1992.

Hardy L; "A Single Judgement Test for Red-Green Discrimination"; *Journal of the Optical Society of America*; Vol 33 9; 1943.

Hayakawa SI; *The Use and Misuse of Language*; Fawcett Pub. Inc.; Greenwich, CT; 1966.

Hayslip B, McBride PA, Lowman RL, Aronson HJ; "Color Vision Deficit and Rorscharch Performance in Aged Persons"; *International Journal of Aging and Human Development*; 34(2):165-73; 1992.

Hering L; *Outline of a Theory of Light and Sense;* Translated by L. Hurvich and D. Jameson; Harvard University Press; Cambridge, MA; 1990.

Hess RF, Sharp LT, Nordby K; *Night Vision: Basic, Clinical and Applied Aspects;* Cambridge University Press; Cambridge, UK; 1990.

Hofstater, DR; *Metamagical Themas: Questing for the Essence of Mind and Pattern;* Basic Books; New York; 1985.

Hopkins C; "Human Factors Mess"; *Machine Design Magazine;* 1:20:83 p4.

Horgan S; "Colorblindness is not a Black and White Rerun of Life"; *San Francisco Chronicle;* April 10, 1986.

Hothersall D; *History of Psychology;* Temple University Press, Philadelphia; p. 55–56; 1984.

Howard D; *Cognitive Psychology: Memory Language and Thought;* MacMillan, NY; 1983.

Hurvich L; "Color Vision and its Deficiences"; *Impact of Science on Society;* Vol. 31 No. 2; p151-164; 1981.

Hurvich L, Jameson D; "Evaluation of Single Pigment Shifts in Anomalous Color Vision"; *Sepataum;* S. Karger; Basel, Switzerland; 1973.

Hurvich L, Jameson D; *The Perception of Brightness and Darkness;* Allyson & Bacon Inc.; Boston, MA; 1966.

IBM; *Human Factors of Work Stations With Visual Displays;* San Jose, CA; 1984.

Ishihara Test; Kanehera & Co. Ltd; Tokyo, Japan; 1994 edition.

Jaeger W, Krastel H, Braun S; "Cerebral Acromatopsia"; *Klinische Monatsblatter Fur Augenheilkunde;* 194(1): 32-6; 1989.

Jaeger W: "Diagnosis of Dominant Infantile Optic Atrophy in Early Childhood"; *Opthalmic Pediatrics and Genetics;* Vol 9, No.1 7-11; 1988.

Jameson D; "Christine Ladd-Franklin"; *Notable American Women 1670-1950 A Biographical Dictionary* Vol II; Belknap Press of Harvard University Press; Cambridge, MA; 354-356; 1971.

Jameson D, Hurvich L; "Intermitent Illumination and Color Vision Testing"; *Mod. Prob. in Opthalmology;* Vol 13; p56-63; S. Karger; Basel, Switzerland; 1973.

Johnson CA, Adams AJ, Casson EJ, Brandt JD; "Progression of Early Glaucomatous Visual Field Loss as Detected by Blue-on-Yellow and Standard White on White Automated Perimetry"; *Arch Opthalmol;* p 651-6; May 1993.

Johnson D; "The Ishihara Test: on the prevention of job discrimination"; *Journal of American Optomentric Association;* 62:352-60; 1992.

Jordan C, Mollon JD; "A Study of Heterozygous Women for Color Deficiencies"; *Vision Research;* Vol. 33 No. II; 1495-1508; 1993.

Judd D, Wyszecki G; *Color in Business Science and Industry;* John Wiley and Sons; NY; 1975.

Kapitansky T, Dietzel M, Grunberger F, Koppelsteiner L, Schleifer G, Max B; "Color Vision Deficiencies in the Course of Acute Alcohol Withdrawl"; *Bio Psychiatry;* Vol 33; 415-422; 1993.

Kidder T; *The Soul of A New Machine;* Avon Books; NY; 1981.

Kock W; *Lasers and Holography: An Introduction to Coherent Optics;* Doubleday; NY; 1969.

Koffka K; *Principles of Gestalt;* Harcourt;

NY; 1935,1963.

Kreifeldt, E; "Optical Method for Screening Diabetes Doesn't Draw Blood"; *Optics and Photonics News*; 8; June, 1995.

Kueppers H; *The Law of Color Theory*; Barrows Educational Series; NY; 1982.

Kueppers H; *Color Atlas*; Barrows Educational Series; NY 1982.

Land E; "The Retinex Theory of Color Vision"; *Scientific American*; December, 1977.

Lefferts R; *Elements of Graphics*; Harper and Row; NY; 1981.

Leonardo Da Vinci; an Artabas Book; Reynal and Co; NY; 1985.

LeSage J, Chuman M; "Color Vision Tests to Identify Elevated Digoxin Levels"; *Research in Nursing and Health*; 9/171-177; 1986.

Lewis PH; "Sorting Out the Graphic Alphabet"; *The New York Times* Sunday Business Section; p.9; May 28, 1988.

Lewis R ed; *Hazardous Chemicals Desk Reference*; Van Nostrand Reinhold; NY; 1991.

Lezheng W; "Hereditary Characteristics of Enzyme Deficiency and Dermatoglyphics in Congenital Color Blindness"; *Japan Opthalmological Journal*; Vol 32:236-245; 1988.

Lide D ed; *Handbook of Chemistry and Physics*; 7th edition; CRC Press; Boca Raton, FL; 1993-4.

Light and Color in the Open Air; 1990 Technical Digest Series; Vol 12; Optical Society of America; Washington, DC; 1990.

Linksz A; "A Short Primer on Color Vision and its Defects"; *Journal of Pedi-atrics*; Vol 5 No 3; Aug, 1969.

Lunardini C; *What Every American Should Know About Women's History*; 165-167; Bob Adams Inc; Hollbrook, MA; 1994.

Luscher M; *The Luscher Color Test*; Random House; NY; 1969.

Lythgroe JN; *The Ecology of Vision*; Claredon Press; Oxford England; 1979.

Mandola J: "Validating the Mandola Test"; *Journal for the Study of Prevention*; Vol 18 p15-18; Spring, 1983.

Mantyjarvi M, Nousiainen IST, Myohaned T; "Color Vision in Diabetic School Children"; *Journal of Ped Opthal and Starb*; Vol 5 No. 5 244-248; 1988.

Marcus A; "Recommended Reading: Workstation Design"; *Computer Graphics Today*; July, 1987.

Marr D; *Vision*; WH Freeman; 1982.

Marre M, Marre E, Harrer S; "Farbesehen bei Katarakt, Aphakie und Pseudophakie", Klin Mbl Augenbleilk; 192:208-215; 1988.

Marzio P; "The Men and Machines of American Journalism"; Smithsonian Institution.

McGuinness D; *When Children Don't Learn*; Basic Books; 1985.

Mc Morrow E; "Lighting Consultants Seek Earlier Role in Design"; *Contract*; January, 1988.

Meads J; "Friendly or Frivolous?"; *Datamation*; p96-100; April, 1985.

Mergler D, Bain L, Lagace JP; "Solvent Related Color Vision Loss: An Indicator of Neural Damage?"; *Occupational and Environmental Health*; Springer Verlag; 1987.

Miller J; *States of Mind*; Pantheon Books; NY; 1983.

Minnaert M; *The Nature of Light and Color in the Open Air*; Dover Publishers Inc; NY; 1954.

Minsky M; *Society of the Mind*; Simon and Shuster; NY; 1986.

Moellering H ed; *Issues in Digital Cartographic Standards*; Report #3; Ohio State University; Columbus, OH.

Motulsky AG; "Normal and Abnormal Color Vision Genes"; *American Journal of Human Genetics*; 42:405-407; 1988.

Munsell AH; *The Grammar of Color*; Strathmore Paper Co.; NY; 1921.

Murch G; "The Effective Use of Color In Graphics"; Proceedings of National Computer Graphics Association Conference; San Jose, CA; p 264-296; 1988.

Nathans J; "The Genes for Color Vision"; *Scientific American*; p42-49; February, 1989.

Nathans J, Davenport CM, Maumenee IH, Lewis RA, Hejtmancik JF, Litt M, Loverien E, Weleber R, Bachynski B, Zwas F, et al; "Molecular Genetics of Human Blue Cone Monochromy"; *Science*; 831-8; Aug, 1989.

Nebette C.B.; *Photography Principles and Practice*; Van Nostrand Co; 1927.

Neitz M, Neitz J; "Numbers and Ratios of Visual Pigment Genes of Normal Red-Green Color Vision"; *Science*; Vol 267; 1013-1016; Feb 17, 1995; .

Notingham N; "Colorblind Machines Slow Holiday Mail"; *Billings Gazette*; p 1; Dec 14, 1994.

Ostroff E ed; *Pioneers of Photography*; Northwestern University Press; 1987.

Pareke S ed; *Dictionary of Scientific Terms*; Fifth Edition; McGraw Hill; New York; 1994.

Pease P, Allen J; "A New Test For Screening Color Vision: Concurrent Validity and Unity"; *American Journal of Optometry and Physiological Optics*; Vol 65, No 9, 729-738; 1988.

Perkins D; *The Mind's Best Work*; Harvard University Press; Cambridge, MA; 1981.

Peters T; "Humanizing Our Companies"; *Electronic Engineering Times*; p96; 7.13; 1984.

Physicians Handbook; Charles E. Baker Co.; 1981.

Pinkers A; "Chromatopsia"; *Documenta Opthalmogica*; 72; 385-390; 1989.

Pledge HT; *Science Since 1500*; Philosophical Library; NY; 1947.

Polakoff P; "Color Blindness is Problem in Some Jobs"; *Northern California Labor*; p 6; June, 1987.

Pokorny J, Smith V; "Eye Disease and Color Defects"; *Vision Res*; Vol 26, No. 9; 1573-1584; 1986.

Pokorny J, Smith V, Verriest G, and Pinkers A; *Congential and Acquired Color Vision Defects*; Grune and Stratton Inc; NY; 1979.

Rochester JB, Gantz J; *The Naked Computer*; William Morrow Inc.; NY; 1983.

Rock I, Palmer S; "The Legacy of Gestalt Psychology"; *Scientific American*; 84-90; December, 1990.

Rood OE; *Modern Chromatics*; Van Nostrand Reinhold Co. NY; 1879, reprint 1973.

Rosenthal O; "Color Blindness and the Computer Industry"; Proceedings of Compint 1985: Canadian Computer

Technologies Conference; Montreal, Canada; p.172-6; 1985.

Rosenthal O; "Color Confusion"; *Optics & Photonics News;* Vol.5 No 7; P8-13; July, 1994.

Rosenthal O; "Grabbing the Eye and Fueling the Mind"; Proceedings of International p 257–262; Computer Color Graphics Conference; Tallahassee FL; 1983.

Roth A, Pellizone M, Hermes D, Sommerhalder J; "Neure Uberlegungen und Entwicklungen zur klinischen Untersuchung des Farbensehens-die Zwei Gleichungsmethode"; *Opttahlmologie;* Springer Verlag; 1989.

Roy MS, Rogers G, Gunkel R, et al; "Color Vision Defects in Sickle Cell Anemia"; *Arch Opthalmol;* 105 1676-1678; 1987.

Rubin L; *Optometry Handbook;* Butterworth Publishers; 1981.

Rushton W.A.H; "Visual Pigments and Color Blindness"; *Scientific American;* p64-9; March, 1975.

Sacks O; *An Anthropologist on Mars; Seven Paradoxical Tales;* Alfred A. Knopf Inc.; NY; 1994.

Scheifer U, Kurtenbach A, Braun E, Kraus W, Zenner E; "Centrally Tinted Contact Lenses: A Useful Aid for Patients With Achromatopsia"; *German Journal of Opthalmology;* 4:52-56; 1995.

Scott I; *The Luscher Color Test;* Pocket Books; NY; 1971.

Seiderman A, Marcus S; *20/20 Is Not Enough;* Alfred A. Knopf Inc.; NY; p97-106; 1989.

Sellers KL, Chioram GM, Dain SJ, Benes SC, Lubow M, Raymohan K, King-Smith PE; "Red Green Mixture Thresholds in Congenital and Acquired Color Vision Defects"; *Vision Res.;* Vol 26; pp 1083-1097; 1986.

Shearson G; "Color Vision Deficiency in Primary School Children"; *Sight Saving Review;* 148-150; Fall, 1965.

Shevell S; "On Neural Signals that Mediate Induced Blackness"; *Vision Res;* Vol 29, No 7, p 891-900; Pergamon Press; 1989.

Shute DT, Oshinskiel L; "Acquired Color Vision Defects and Self-monitoring of Blood Sugar in Diabetes"; *J Amer Opth Assoc;* 57, 824-831; 1986.

Sibert J; "Interactive Specifications of Color For Time Series Mapping"; Proceedings of Harvard Computer Graphics Conference; Cambridge, MA; 1982.

Sizer N; *Heads and Faces and How to Study Them: A Manual of Phrenology and Physiognomy for the People;* Fowler and Wells Co.; NY; 1892.

Sloane P; *The Visual Nature of Color;* Design Press; NY; 1989.

Sobel R; *The Manipulators;* Anchor Press/Doubleday; Garden City; NY; 1976.

Somerfield M, Long G, Porter T, Gillard E: "Effects of Viewing Conditions on Standard Measures of Acquired and Congenital Color Defects"; *Optometry and Vision Science;* Vol 66, No 1 p 29-33; 1989.

Stix G; "Stained Glass"; *Scientific American;* p 118; June, 1992.

Steward JM , Cole B; "What Do Color Vision Defectives Say About Everyday Tasks?"; *Optometry and Vision Science;* Vol 66, No.5; 288-295; 1989.

Stroop JR; "Studies of Inference in Serial Verbal Reactions"; *Journal of Experi-*

mental Psychology; 18:643-662; 1935.

Strutt JW; *The Collected Papers of Lord Rayleigh;* Vol I; Part A: 595-596, Part B: 776-784, 844-853, 999-1005, 1203-1204; Optical Society of America; Washington, DC; 1994.

Swanson WH, Everett M; "Color Vision Screening of Young Children"; *Journal of Opthalmic Nursing & Technology;* 11(4):164-71; July-Aug, 1992.

Swezey R, Davis E; "A Case Study of Human Factors"; *Guidelines in Computer Graphics; IEEE;* p 21-25; Nov, 1983.

Trzcinski J, Stepie J, Berner B; "Disorder of Color Vision in Employees of the Masovian Refining and Petrochemical Industries in Poland"; *Klinika Oczna;* 91(2-3):43-4; Feb-Mar, 1989.

Vreese L; "Two System for Colour-Naming Defect: Verbal Disconnection vs Colour Imagery Disorder"; *Neuropsychologia;* Vol 29; No 1 1-18; 1991.

Vyngrys A, Cole B; "Are Colour Vision Standards Justified for the Transport Industry?"; *British Opthal Physiol Opt;* Vol 8; 257-272; July, 1988.

Wertbenbaker L; *The Eye: Window to the World;* US News Books; Washington, DC; 1981.

Wilkinson W; "The Cognitive and Social Emotional Correlates of Color Deficiency in Children"; paper presented at the annual meeting of the Arizona Educational Research Associa-

tion; Pheonix, AZ; 1990.

Wilson G; *Researches in Colour Blindness: With a Supplement on the Danger Attending the Present System of Railway and Marine Coloured Signals;* Southerland & Knox; Edinburgh; 1855.

Widengard I, Mandahl A, Tornquist P, Wistrand PJ; "Colour Vision and Side Effects During Treatment with Methazolamide"; *Eye;* p 130–135. 9/1995

Wright A, Barry J ed; *Molecular Genetics of Inherited Eye Disorders;* p 217-257; Harwood Academic Publishers; GmbH; 1994.

Wurman R; *Follow The Yellow Brick Road;* Bantam Books; NY; 1992.

Yahoo and Lycros Search catalog 10797133 unique URLs on the World Wide Web under *colorblind.*

Yeh T, Smith V, Pokorny J; "The Effect of Background Luminance on Cone Sensitivity Functions"; *Investigative Opthalmology and Visual Science;* Vol 30/10; October, 1989.

Zentall S; "Attention Cuing in Spelling Tasks for Hyperactive and Comparison Regular Classroom Children"; *Journal of Special Education;* Vol 23 83-93; Spring, 1989.

Also:

Countless interviews with and communications from colorblind people.

Suggested Reading

Alberti, R., Emmons, R. *Your Perfect Right*. San Luis Obispo, CA: Impact Press, 1974

Barker, L. *Listening Behavior*. Englewood Cliffs, NJ: Prentice-Hall, 1971

Benson, H. *The Relaxation Response*. New York: Morrow, 1975

Bloch, D. *Words That Heal*. New York: Bantam, 1990

Bloomer, C.M. *Principles of Visual Perception*. New York: Van Nostrand Reinhold Co, 1976

Bower, S., Bower, G. *Asserting Yourself*. Reading, MA: Addison-Wesley, 1976

Bry, A. *Friendship, How To Have A Friend And Be A Friend*. New York: Grosset Dunlap, 1979

Burns, D. *Feeling Good*. New York: Signet, 1981

Burns, D. *The Feeling Good Handbook*. New York: William Morrow, 1989

DePaulo, J., Ablow, K. *How to Cope With Depression*. New York: McGraw-Hill, 1989

Goethe, W. *Color Study*. Cambridge, MA: MIT Press, 1982

Goulding, M. *Not To Worry! How To Free Yourself From Unnecessary Anxiety And Channel Your Worries Into Positive Action*. New York: Silver Arrow/William Morrow, 1989

Helmstetter, S. *What To Say When You Talk to Yourself*. New York: Pocket Books, 1982

Kushner, H. *When Bad Things Happen To Good People*. New York: Avon, 1981

Lieberman, M., Hardie, M. *Resolving Family and Other Conflicts*. Santa Cruz, CA: Unity, 1981

Mason, J. *Guide To Stress Reduction.* Berkeley, CA: Celestial Arts, 1985

Sacks, O. *The Island of the Colorblind.* New York: Alfred Knopf, 1997

Sloane, P. *The Visual Nature of Color.* New York: Design Press, 1989

Walton, D. *Are You Communicating? You Can't Manage Without It.* New York: McGraw-Hill, 1989

Weekes, C. *Hope and Help For Your Nerves.* New York: Bantam, 1978

Wolpe, J., Wolpe, D. *Life Without Fear.* Oakland: New Harbinger, 1988

Yapko, M. *Free Yourself From Depression.* Emmaus, PA: Rodale Press, 1992

Index